# CLINICAL PSYCHOPHARMACOLOGY

**made
ridiculously
simple**

John Preston, Psy.D., ABPP
*Alliant International University*
*Sacramento, California*

James Johnson, M.D.
*Kaiser Medical Center*
*Department of Psychiatry*
*South Sacramento, California*

ISBN 10# 1-935660-05-5
ISBN 13# 978-1-935660-05-7

*Made in the United States of America*


Published by
MedMaster, Inc.
P.O. Box 640028
Miami, Fla.  33164

*For Bonnie and Mary*

# Contents

# Preface

This brief book provides an overview of clinical psychopharmacology. Successful medical treatment of emotional and mental disorders depends on two factors: a thorough knowledge of psychotropic medications and an accurate diagnosis. Both issues are addressed in this book in a practical and concise format.

To the best of our knowledge, recommended doses for medications listed in this book are accurate. However, they are not meant to serve as a guide for prescription of medications. Please check the manufacturer's product information sheet or the *Physicians' Desk Reference* for any changes in dosage schedule or contraindications.

We wish to express our appreciation to the following people who have reviewed this book and made a number of helpful suggestions: John H. Greist, M.D., Donald Klein, M.D., Glen Hakanson, M.D., and Patrick Donlon, M.D. Many thanks to Michelle Riekstins for her help in the preparation of the manuscript and to our editor, Dr. Stephen Goldberg, for many helpful suggestions.

# Chapter 1   General Principles

## BIOLOGY vs. PSYCHOLOGY

For many years a debate raged in psychiatry with regard to the etiology and treatment of major mental disorders. Two opposing camps emerged: biological psychiatry, whose devotees held that psychiatric disorders had an organic basis; and psychologically oriented psychiatry, probably best represented by the psychodynamic movement, whose converts focused on the role of current emotional stressors, early childhood traumas, interpersonal problems, and intrapsychic conflict as causal agents in the development of psychiatric symptomatology. Although these polar views still exist, in recent years there has been an emerging view that encompasses both psychological and physiological factors in the etiology and treatment of many psychiatric disorders. In many, if not most, mental disorders it is helpful to think of a continuum or spectrum. Almost all mental disorders usually represent heterogeneous syndromes.

When one talks about depression, for instance, it is important to realize that depression can present in a number of different ways and may have diverse etiologies. In some instances the cause may be purely psychological, e.g., a reaction to losing a job, death of a loved one, a significant rejection, etc. Likewise, symptoms may be largely psychological, e.g., feelings of low self-esteem and sadness. In other cases the picture is one of a pure biological disorder which has little or no connection to environmental precipitants, but rather involves an endogenous neurochemical malfunction. In addition to psychological symptoms, the resulting symptoms may include a host of somatic symptoms, such as sleep disturbance and weight loss. Clearly, in some individuals there is an interplay of environmental/psychological factors *and* biochemical dysfunctions. The question "Is this a psychological or biological problem?" is overly simplistic. Rather, one must ask, "To what extent is this disorder due to psychological factors and to what extent is it due to a biochemical disturbance?" The answer to this question is extremely important in guiding treatment decisions. *Most purely psychological problems are not helped by medication treatment. On the other hand, most biologically based psychiatric disorders require medication treatment.*

In this book we hope to provide key diagnostic guidelines to help the clinician pinpoint the diagnosis and develop a realistic treatment plan.

# Chapter 2 Depression

## DIAGNOSIS

### Major Clinical Features and Differential Diagnosis

It is important to distinguish between (1) reactive sadness, (2) grief, (3) medical illness and medications that cause depressive symptoms, (4) clinical depression (also commonly referred to as unipolar or major depression), and (5) dysthymia. The first two are painful but normal emotional reactions and usually do not require treatment. These four syndromes may be distinguished by the following characteristics:

1. *Reactive Sadness.* The emotional reaction stems from a relatively minor event. It is transient (a few hours to a few days) and rarely interferes with functioning.

2. *Grief.* This is a normal response to a major interpersonal loss (such as the death of a loved one or marital separation/divorce). This experience can be tremendously painful and is much more prolonged than reactive sadness. Please note that "normal" grief can last for many months and it is not uncommon for noticeable sadness and loneliness to persist for several years following significant interpersonal losses. Grief differs from clinical depression in four ways:

   a. Despite intense sadness, there is no significant loss of self-esteem.

   b. Markers that grief has developed into clinical depression include: severe sleep disturbances (especially early morning awakening), a pervasive loss of interest in normal life activities, significant agitation, and/or suicidal ideations.

   c. The patient clearly relates the sadness to the loss. There may be active mourning and pining for the loved one; the painful feelings "make sense."

   d. Grief work (i.e., mourning) and time are often the major ingredients necessary for emotional healing.
   Note that at least 25% of people experiencing a major loss will initially exhibit grief reactions, but during the year following the loss will go on to develop major depression. Additionally, 10% of bereaved individuals will develop traumatic stress symptoms following interpersonal losses (e.g.. intense anxiety, nightmares). Thus one must have a high index of suspicion for these common forms of complicated bereavement.

3. *Medical Illnesses and Medications That Can Cause Depression.* Certain medical disorders (see Figure 1) can at times result in biochemical changes

that affect central neurotransmitters, thereby triggering serious depressive reactions. Hypothyroidism (especially subclinical presentations) is clearly the most common medical disorder causing depressive symptoms (accounting for 5-10% of major depressions), thus it is always important to screen for thyroid disease. Likewise, some medications can cause depression as a side effect (see Figure 2). Please note that minor tranquilizers may cause or exacerbate depression. A very frequent treatment mistake is for the physician to be impressed by the more obvious symptoms of anxiety or agitation, to fail to recognize an underlying depression, and to only prescribe a benzodiazepine/minor tranquilizer. (Note: 50% of cases of major depression are accompanied by significant anxiety or agitation) The result is often some initial calming, but after a few weeks the depression worsens. If the basic disorder is depression, but with coexisting anxiety symptoms, it is important to treat the depression. With appropriate treatment for the depression, the anxiety symptoms will generally subside.

It is very important to note that it is common during periods of depression for patients to significantly increase their use of caffeine. Caffeine of course combats fatigue, but it also has mild, transient antidepressant actions, and thus people gravitate towards increasing use. This results in a commonly overlooked complication to treatment: caffeine amounts in excess of 250 mg. per day can contribute to a decrease in slow wave (deep) sleep; slow wave sleep is already decreased in depression and the further erosion of this form of restorative sleep often worsens depression. Caffeine also contributes to restless sleep and frequent awakenings during the night. It is important for patients to know that this effect can occur even in the absence of initial insomnia. This is such a pervasive problem that it is essential to take a caffeine history on *all* patients suffering from psychiatric disorders (please see Appendix C for a brief caffeine questionnaire). With depression every attempt should be made to keep caffeine consumption below 250 mg a day (and preferably used only in the morning). Many patients will not take such recommendations seriously unless the physician makes a point to explain its impact on sleep.

When the basic cause of depression is one of the illnesses listed in Figure 1 or a side effect of medication, the primary focus should be on treating the core illness or switching medications. When such interventions are carried out, the depression will usually lift.

4. *Clinical Depression.* This is a pathological process characterized as follows:

   a. Depressed mood (sadness or emptiness) or irritability is often continuous and pervasive.

   b. A loss of interest in normal life activities.

   c. There is increasing impairment of normal functioning (work, school, and intimate relationships).

   d. There is an irrational or exaggerated erosion of self-esteem.

*Figure 1*

## COMMON DISORDERS THAT MAY CAUSE DEPRESSION

- Addison's disease
- AIDS
- Alzheimer's disease
- Anemia
- Apnea
- Asthma
- Chronic Fatigue Syndromes
- Chronic infection (mononucleosis, TB)
- Chronic pain
- Congestive heart failure
- Cushing's disease
- Diabetes
- Hyperthyroidism
- Hypothyroidism
- Infectious Hepatitis

- Influenza
- Malignancies (cancer)
- Malnutrition
- Menopause
- Multiple sclerosis
- Parkinson's disease
- Post-partum hormonal changes
- Porphyria
- Premenstrual syndrome
- Rheumatoid arthritis
- Syphilis
- Systemic lupus erythematosis
- Ulcerative colitis
- Uremia
- Lyme disease

   e. There is a dramatic and specific change in vegetative patterns (e.g., sleep, appetite, sex drive, etc.) and the appearance of nonspecific physical complaints.

   f. Depression can occur in response to psychological stressors, or may emerge without clear-cut precipitating events.

5. *Dysthymia:* low-grade, chronic depression. Long-standing dysphoria, irritability, low-self-esteem and often a lack of enthusiasm. This condition is less severe than clinical depression and typically does not interfere with daily functioning.

## Target Symptoms

All types of depression tend to share certain universal symptoms (see Figure 3). Disorders that reflect an underlying biochemical dysfunction typically present with *both* the universal symptoms *and* the physiological symptoms (Figure 4).

# ANTIDEPRESSANT MEDICATION

## When Do You Prescribe Antidepressants?

The most important guideline for prescribing antidepressant medication is whether or not there are sustained physiological symptoms, as outlined below (see Figure 4). Occasional disturbances of sleep or appetite, for instance, do not warrant

*Figure 2*

**DRUGS THAT MAY CAUSE DEPRESSION**

| TYPE | GENERIC NAME | BRAND NAME |
|------|--------------|------------|
| ■ *Antihypertensives* (for high blood pressure) | reserpine | Serpasil, Ser-Ap-Es, Sandril |
| | propranolol hydrochloride | Inderal |
| | methyldopa | Aldomet |
| | guanethidine sulfate | Ismelin sulfate |
| | clonidine hydrochloride | Catapres |
| | hydralazine hydrochloride | Apresoline hydrochloride |
| ■ *Corticosteroids and other Hormones* | cortisone acetate | Cortone |
| | estrogen | Evex, Menrium, Femest |
| | progesterone and derivatives | Lipo-Lutin, Progestasert, Proluton |
| | prednisone | Various Brands |
| ■ *Antiparkinson Drugs* | levodopa and carbidopa | Sinemet |
| | levodopa | Dopar, Larodopa |
| | amantadine hydrochloride | Symmetrel |
| ■ *Antianxiety Drugs* | diazepam and others | Valium (see Figure 21) |
| ■ *Birth Control Pills* | progesterone estrogen | Various Brands |
| ■ *Alcohol* | wine, beer, spirits | Various Brands |
| ■ *Antibiotics* | ribavirin, interferons | Various Brands |

*Figure 3*

**SYMPTOMS COMMON TO ALL DEPRESSIONS**

- ■ Mood of sadness, despair, emptiness
- ■ Anhedonia (loss of the ability to experience pleasure and a loss of interest in normal life activities)[1]
- ■ Low self-esteem
- ■ Apathy, low motivation, and social withdrawal

- ■ Excessive emotional sensitivity
- ■ Negative, pessimistic thinking
- ■ Irritability and low frustration tolerance
- ■ Suicidal ideas
- ■ Excessive guilt
- ■ Indecisiveness

[1]*Note:* Some degree of decreased capacity for pleasure may be seen in all types of depression. In severe depressions and in those that involve a biochemical disturbance, this loss of ability to experience pleasure can become so pronounced that the patient has almost no moments of joy or pleasure. Such people are said to have a "non-reactive mood," which means that they are unable to temporarily get out of their depressed mood.

*Figure 4*

**VEGETATIVE/PHYSIOLOGICAL SYMPTOMS REFLECTING
A BIOCHEMICAL DYSFUNCTION**
(PRIMARY TARGET SYMPTOMS FOR MEDICATION TREATMENT)

- Sleep disturbance (early morning awakening, decreased sleep efficiency, frequent awakenings throughout the night,[1] occasionally hypersomnia: excessive sleeping)
- Appetite disturbance (decreased or increased, with accompanying weight loss or gain)
- Fatigue
- Decreased sex drive
- Restlessness, agitation, or psychomotor retardation
- Diurnal variations in mood (usually feeling worse in the morning)
- Impaired concentration and forgetfulness
- Pronounced anhedonia (total loss of the ability to experience pleasure)

---

[1]*Note:* Initial insomnia (difficulty in falling asleep) may be seen with depression but is not diagnostic of a major depressive disorder. Initial insomnia can be seen in anyone experiencing stress in general. Initial insomnia alone is more characteristic of anxiety disorders than of depression.

medication treatment. However, if there is continuing weight loss, marked fatigue each day, and poor sleep most nights, antidepressants are indicated. In the Appendix we have included a brief symptom checklist that can be used to quickly assess a host of psychiatric symptoms. Depressive symptoms are included under Section A. Additionally, those patients who are depressed and are judged to be poor psychotherapy candidates (e.g., lower intelligence, not psychologically minded, or those who refuse psychotherapy) should be considered for a trial on antidepressants.

## Choosing Medication

Antidepressant medications fall into two primary groups: (1) typical antidepressants, and (2) MAO inhibitors. Empirical studies suggest that certain symptomatic presentations may point toward preferred first-line medication choices. This has resulted in the development of treatment guidelines. If the clinical picture is dominated by: anxiety, agitation, obsessional symptoms, rumination, irritability, aggression, and/or pronounced suicidality, serotonin reuptake inhibitors are the first-line treatment strategy (see Figure 5: those drugs indicated with an *). If the clinical picture is characterized by: apathy, low energy, anhedonia, and/or low motivation, dopamine or noradrenergic reuptake inhibitors are preferred (e.g., bupropion). (NIMH, 2002; Goodwin and Jamison, 2007)

A second major factor in choosing an antidepressant is the side effect profile (side effects are described in figure 5 and on page 12).

*Figure 5*

## ANTIDEPRESSANT MEDICATIONS

| GENERIC | BRAND | USUAL DAILY DOSAGE RANGE | SEDATION | ACH EFFECTS[1] |
|---|---|---|---|---|
| *TYPICAL ANTIDEPRESSANTS* | | | | |
| imipramine | Tofranil | 150–300 mg | mid | mid |
| desipramine | Norpramin | 150–300 mg | low | low |
| amitriptyline | Elavil | 150–300 mg | high | high |
| nortriptyline | Aventyl, Pamelor | 75–125 mg | mid | mid |
| protriptyline | Vivactil | 15–40 mg | low | mid |
| trimipramine | Surmontil | 100–300 mg | high | mid |
| doxepin | Sinequan, Adapin | 150–300 mg | high | mid |
| maprotiline | Ludiomil | 150–225 mg | mid | low |
| amoxapine | Asendin | 150–400 mg | mid | low |
| trazodone | Desyrel[2] | 150–400 mg | mid | none |
| fluoxetine* | Prozac, Sarafem | 20–80 mg | low | none |
| bupropion, S.R. | Wellbutrin, S.R. | 150–300 mg | low | none |
| sertraline* | Zoloft | 50–200 mg | low | none |
| paroxetine* | Paxil | 20–50 mg | low | low |
| venlafaxine, X.R. | Effexor, X.R. | 75–350 mg | low | none |
| desvenlafaxine | Pristiq | 50–300 mg | low | none |
| nefazodone | Serzone[2] | 100–500 mg | mid | low |
| fluvoxamine* | Luvox | 50–300 mg | low | low |
| mirtazapine | Remeron | 15–45 mg | mid | mid |
| citalopram* | Celexa | 10–60 mg | low | none |
| escitalopram* | Lexapro | 5–20 mg | low | none |
| duloxetine | Cymbalta | 20–80 mg | low | none |
| atomoxetine | Strattera | 60–120 mg | low | low |
| vilazodone | Viibryd | 10–40 mg | low | none |
| *MAO INHIBITORS[3]* | | | | |
| phenelzine | Nardil | 30–90 mg | low | none |
| tranylcypromine | Parnate | 20–60 mg | low | none |
| isocarboxazid | Marplan | 10–40 mg | low | none |
| selegiline | Emsam | 6–12 mg | low | none |

[1]*ACH EFFECTS* (anticholinergic side effects) include dry mouth, constipation, difficulty in urinating, and blurry vision. Can cause confusion and memory disturbances in the elderly or brain-damaged patient.

[2]Due to short half-life, requires divided dosing. The brand name drug Serzone is no longer being manufactured.

[3]Require strict adherence to dietary and medication regimen. Emsam at a dose of 6 mg does not require dietary restrictions.

*Note:* Prescribe maprotiline and bupropion to patients with history of seizures only with great caution.

*A widely prescribed class of antidepressants are the *selective serotonin reuptake inhibitors* (SSRIs), which include: fluoxetine, paroxetine, sertraline, fluvoxamine, citalopram, and escitalopram.

## Prescribing Treatment

Antidepressant medications are generally started at a low dosage and gradually titrated up. With depressed patients even slight side effects often lead to non-compliance. The most common mistake made by family physicians is to under-medicate. Although there are exceptions, generally a patient (ages 16–55) must receive a dose that is within the therapeutic range (see Figure 5). (Doses for those over 55 are often somewhat lower.)

Typical start-up regimes would be as follows:

| Drug | (doses for adults ages 16-55) Starting dose | Increase in 1-2 weeks, if tolerated |
|------|---------------------------------------------|-------------------------------------|
| Fluoxetine | 10 mg | 20 mg |
| Sertraline | 50 mg | 100 mg |
| Paroxetine | 10 mg | 20 mg |
| Citalopram | 20 mg | 40 mg |
| Venlafaxine, XR | 37.5 mg bid | 75 mg bid |
| Desvenlafaxine | 50 mg | 50–100 mg |
| Bupropion, SR | 100 mg | 100 mg bid |
| Nefazodone | 50 mg bid | 100 mg bid |
| Mirtazapine | 15 mg | 30 mg |
| Escitalopram | 5 mg | 10 mg |
| Duloxetine | 20 mg | 40 mg |
| Atomoxetine | 25 mg | 60 mg |
| Vilazodone | 10 mg | 20–30 mg |

Increases in dose can be made if there is a failure to show a positive response after 4–5 weeks of treatment. Note: If the patient had first episode prior to the age of 18, is experiencing a recurrent episode, and/or has been depressed for more than two months, this often requires 4–6 weeks to show first signs of a clinical response.

The treatment of major depression involves three phases:

*Acute Treatment:* Begins with the first dose and extends until the patient is asymptomatic (in good case scenarios, this may be from 6–8 weeks but often takes longer).

*Continuation Treatment:* To avoid acute relapse, it is strongly suggested that patients continue treatment for a minimum of six months beyond the acute phase. Also, recent studies indicate that the patient should be maintained on the *same* dose used during the acute phase.

*Maintenance Treatment:* Relapse prevention is an important aspect of treatment, especially in those patients judged to have recurrent episodes (or at risk for recurrence).* Continued (lifelong) treatment provides the best outcome for such

*Note:* 70–80% of patients with major depression will experience either chronic or recurrent, episodic depressions.

## *Figure 6*

### DECISION TREE FOR DIAGNOSIS
### AND TREATMENT OF DEPRESSION - I

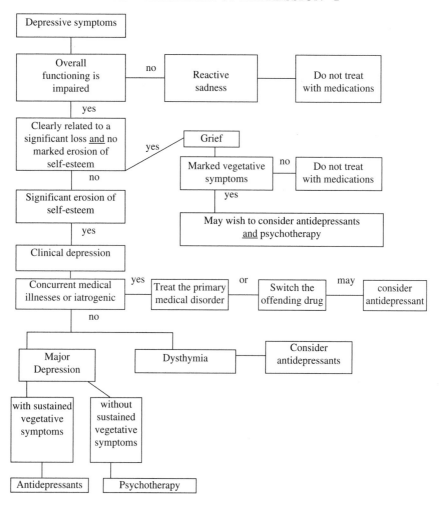

individuals. Chronic treatment may protect many individuals from subsequent episodes, although most patients suffering from recurrent major depression will experience some additional episodes (albeit, with decreased frequency and severity). The following guidelines are offered:

1. *First Episode:* At the end of the continuation phase, gradually reduce the dose (over a period of 4–6 weeks to avoid acute discontinuation withdrawal symptoms) and, assuming no return of depressive symptoms, discontinue. Educate the patient to be

*Figure 6 (cont.)*

## DECISION TREE: TREATMENT OF DEPRESSION - II

**Phase of Treatment**

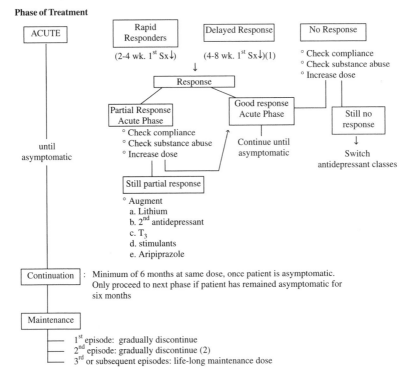

Footnotes:
1. Patients with the following characteristics may ultimately be good responders, but take longer to achieve first signs of symptomatic improvement: current episode has been ongoing for more than three months and the symptoms are severe.
2. If a second episode and these risk factors are present, may consider life-long treatment: first episode was prior to the age of 18, family history of mood disorders, inter-episode the patient was not eu-thymic (i.e., did not fully recover from first episode).
3. This decision tree is based on results from the Texas Medication Algorithm Project (1998) and A. John Rush (1997). Note that the general concepts from the project are addressed in this decision-tree, however, the particular graphics above were developed by the authors of this book.

alert to any signs of recurrence (e.g., poor sleep, fatigue, etc.) and should this oc-cur, contact the treating doctor as soon as possible to reinstigate treatment.

2. *Second Episode:*

   a. With *"Risk Factors"* which include family history of mood disorders, first episode occurring prior to the age of 18, and/or most recent episode has severe symptoms: Recommend life-long medication treatment to prevent recurrence.

   b. Without *"Risk Factors"*: gradually discontinue medications.

3. *Third or later episodes.* Recommend life-long medication treatment.

## Figure 7

## SPECIAL PROBLEMS AND MEDICATIONS OF CHOICE

| THE PROBLEM | MEDICATION CONSIDERATIONS |
|---|---|
| 1. High suicide risk[1] | 1. Avoid tricyclics and MAOIs |
| 2. Concurrent depression and panic attacks or OCD | 2. venlafaxine, SSRIs |
| 3. Chronic pain with or without depression | 3. amitriptyline, doxepin, venlafaxine, duloxetine |
| 4. Weight gain on other antidepressants | 4. bupropion, SSRIs[2] avoid mirtazapine |
| 5. Sensitivity to anticholinergic side effects | 5. Avoid tricyclics and paroxetine |
| 6. Orthostatic hypotension | 6. nortriptyline, bupropion, sertraline |
| 7. Sexual dysfunction | 7. bupropion, nefazodone |

[1]*Note:* Many older-generation antidepressants (e.g. tricyclics and MAO inhibitors) are quite toxic when taken in overdose. Extreme caution should be exercised in prescribing to high-risk suicidal patients.
[2]Weight gain is rare in the acute phase of treatment with SSRIs, however, with prolonged use approximately 10% of patients will experience noticeable weight gain.

## What to Expect

It has been hypothesized that many of the primary symptoms of clinical depression are caused by a dysregulation of certain neurotransmitters (e.g., norepinephrine, dopamine, and/or serotonin) and intracellular second messengers. Antidepressant medications are able to restore normal neurochemical functioning in key limbic structures in the brain. They have also been shown to increase the production of neuroprotective proteins (e.g. BDNF) and reduce levels of stress hormones (e.g. cortisol). It is very important to note, however, that these drugs do not act rapidly. It generally requires 2–4 weeks of treatment for symptoms to *begin* to improve. This is a crucial point. Many, if not most, depressed patients become easily discouraged if there is no relief in a few days. Such patients often discontinue medications prematurely.

## Side Effects

Probably owing to their tremendous feelings of hopelessness and pessimism, depressed patients are especially prone to discontinuing treatment prematurely. This is often the case when they encounter side effects which typically emerge long before the therapeutic effects are realized. Thus, choosing medications that are low in side effects is an important rule of thumb. Fortunately, most newer generation antidepressants have a far better side effect profile than older generation tricyclics. Side effects certainly account for treatment failures, however, it should be noted that other factors also contribute to treatment drop-outs (see Figure 8). It is likely that many drop-outs are due to the prolonged time before the onset of symptomatic improvement and tremendous pessimism that is a cardinal feature of depression.

*Figure 8*

**Drop-outs due to side effects**
**First six weeks of treatment**

| | |
|---|---|
| Placebo | 3–7% |
| Tricyclics | 25–30% |
| New generation antidepressants | 9–21% |

## Side Effect Management Considerations: SSRIs

SSRIs are judged to be very effective medications for the treatment of depression presenting with agitation and/or co-morbid anxiety. However, many patients experience an increase in anxiety, restlessness, and/or insomnia during the first week or two of treatment (i.e. this is referred to as activation and is a common acute side effect which may emerge several hours after taking the first dose of an SSRI or soon after increasing the dose). This side effect can be *very* problematic in that it often leads to patient-initiated discontinuation. Typically this side effect diminishes in 2–3 weeks. An often-effective solution is to begin treatment by co-administering a low dose of a minor tranquilizer (e.g. 0.25–0.5 mg lorazepam, bid or tid) to be used only for the first month of treatment, and then discontinued. This not only controls drug-induced activation but can also provide very quick relief from anxiety if co-morbid anxiety is a part of the clinical picture. The rapid decrease in anxiety is often experienced by the patient as a very positive sign that medication treatments can be helpful and may inspire hope to continue taking medications until the more prominent antidepressant actions begin to emerge. If the only manifestation of activation is initial insomnia, then the use of the sedating antidepressant, trazodone (e.g., 50–75 mg qhs) or mirtazapine (Remeron, 7.5-15 mg qhs) are popular and effective strategies. Trazodone or Remeron are also drugs of choice for initial insomnia in patients where there is a history or suspected problem of substance abuse (they are non-habit-forming).

SSRIs are widely prescribed for depression owing to their effectiveness and relatively low incidence of side effects. Recently, three late-onset side effects (generally seen several months into treatment) have been noted. These side effects are a common reason for patient-initiated discontinuation or poor compliance, and are side effects patients seldom report (thus, it is important for the physician to inquire). Sexual dysfunction (primarily inorgasmia) occurs as a side effect in 25-30% of patients taking SSRIs or other antidepressants that have significant serotonergic actions (i.e. venlafaxine, nefazodone, mirtazapine) (Clayton, et al. 2002). Please note that the base rate for sexual dysfunction (SD) in the general population is rather high and is also a common symptom of depression. Thus various causes of SD are commonly seen in depressed patients (however, the main type of SD seen as an antidepressant *side effect* is inorgasmia). Impotence is rare as a side effect. Interestingly, sildenafil (Viagra), which was developed to treat male erectile dysfunction, has been used successfully to combat drug-induced inorgasmia in both men and women. A second late-onset side effect is decreased spontaneity and apathy. This side effect may be spotted by reports by the patient that "I'm feeling depressed again." However, on closer inspection most depressive symptoms continue to be in remission. Rather, the patient is experiencing either a loss of motivation or a decreased sense of emotional aliveness (sometimes including an inability to cry). The third late-onset side effect is weight gain (which apparently is not associated with increased caloric intake, and affects about 10% of patients on chronic SSRI treatment).

These side effects can often be successfully managed by the solutions indicated below:

*Figure 9*

| PROBLEM | TREATMENT OPTION |
|---|---|
| ■ Inorgasmia | ■ Reduce SSRI dose, or<br>■ Sildenafil (50–100 mg., p.r.n.)<br>■ Add bupropion<br>■ Add cyproheptadine 4–12 mg., p.r.n. |
| ■ Apathy, decreased spontaneity | ■ Reduce SSRI dose, or<br>■ Add bupropion (start low: e.g., 75 mg. b.i.d. and do not exceed 300 mg. q.d.) |
| ■ Weight gain | ■ Exercise and dieting |

## Common Treatment Errors to Avoid

- Under-dosing
- Poor compliance
- Misdiagnosis: especially problematic if the patient actually has bipolar disorder. Antidepressants in bipolar patients may provoke manic episodes and/or increase frequency of episodes.
- Co-morbid substance abuse; especially moderate-to-heavy alcohol use (if not detected, can result in treatment failure of antidepressants. This is a very common reason for inadequate medication response).
- Using benzodiazepines to treat depression (can increase depressive symptoms and may lead to drug dependence/abuse)
- Premature discontinuation
- Rapid discontinuation

# KEY POINTS TO COMMUNICATE TO PATIENTS

In prescribing antidepressant medication, patient education is especially important. Listed below are the key points to communicate to patients starting on antidepressants.

1. Onset of clinical action generally takes 2–4 weeks. It will take this long for you to notice the onset of reduction of symptoms.

2. Symptomatic improvement is usually seen primarily in the physiological symptoms (Figure 4). Many of the other symptoms (e.g., depressed mood, low self-esteem, etc.) may respond only partially to medication treatment. These medications are not "happy pills"; they do not totally erase feelings of sadness or emptiness.

3. The best barometers of early medication response generally include improved sleep, less daytime fatigue, and some improvement in emotional control (e.g., less frequent crying spells or better frustration tolerance). The prescriber may need to inquire specifically about these symptoms because many depressed people will say "I'm no better," despite the fact that there are subtle signs of symptomatic improvement.

4. There may be side effects. However, side effects can most often be managed by dosage adjustment or by switching to another medication.

5. Total length of treatment varies considerably for individuals. Typically, it may take 6–8 weeks for the major depressive symptoms to subside. It is very important not to discontinue treatment at this point. The acute relapse rate can be as high as 50+%. The general rule of thumb is to continue treatment for a period of 6 months beyond the point of symptomatic improvement and then gradually to reduce the dose. Should symptoms return during this medication-reduction phase of treatment, the dosage should again be increased. Medication should be continued for 2–3 months before another trial on lower doses. Occasionally, a person may need to be on long-term chronic medication management.

6. Antidepressants are not addictive.

7. You should not drink alcohol when taking antidepressants. Alcohol can block the effects of the antidepressants (although, in clinical practice, many physicians will allow patients on antidepressants to have an occasional drink, but not in excess of one per day).

8. Never discontinue "cold turkey"; this can result in withdrawal symptoms. Withdrawal symptoms can include nausea, anxiety, insomnia, flu-like general malaise and sometimes a peculiar sensation described by patients as "electrical shocks" experienced in the limbs or the head.

9. Two strategies always improve depression: exercise and a reduction of substances that impair sleep (most common: caffeine and alcohol).

## If First Line Medications Do Not Lead to Remission

Generally it is best to start with a typical antidepressant. It is necessary to treat at adequate doses; most treatment failures are due to inadequate doses. Unless side effects are intolerable or a person is a high-risk patient (see *Precautions,* p. 17), standard practice is to gradually push the dose to the upper level of the therapeutic range until symptomatic improvement is attained. This strategy was borne out in a recent large-scale study (STAR-D program) supported by the National Institute of Mental Health. The best results were achieved beginning with standard doses (see table on page 8). If there was a failure to respond by week four doses were gradually increased (e.g. Celexa: 60 mg.; Effexor: 375 mg; Wellbutrin: 400 mg . . . unless side effects prohibited this). Failure to use high enough dosing is a common reason for lack of response. In this study, those who experienced significant improvement or remission generally did so within 7 weeks. If a patient is on a high dose for a period of 4–6 weeks without symptomatic improvement, it is unlikely that improvement will occur. If there is a partial response, then a strategy that is often successful is to augment. The most common forms of augmentation are: SSRI plus bupropion (e.g. 150-400 mg qd), T3, 25-50 micrograms qd, SSRI plus low dose stimulant (e.g. methylphenidate, 5-10 mg) especially for depressions accompanied by marked fatigue and apathy, buspirone (15-40 mg qd) especially for depressions with co-morbid anxiety symptoms, addition of the antipsychotic aripiprazole (note: this medication has FDA approval for augmenting antidepressant treatment in non-psychotic depressions; it also can treat psychotic depressions), or antidepressant plus low doses of lithium (e.g., 600-900 mg qd). A fairly large number of non-respondents do benefit from augmentation. Should this fail, then a change in the antidepressant medication is in order.

The next step generally is to switch to another typical antidepressant. The choice is guided by two factors: side effect profiles and neurotransmitter action. There is some evidence to suggest that there exist three basic neurochemicals that may be affected in major depressive disorder: norepinephrine, dopamine and serotonin. The various antidepressant medications have different effects on these three neurochemical systems (see Figure 10). Some are considered to have broad spectrum effects ("shotguns") and others are more selective ("bullets"). If your first unsuccessful drug was serotonergic, then the second choice should be a medication targeting norepinephrine or dopamine.

What if this fails too? The next strategy is to switch to mirtazanine, venlafaxine, duloxetine, or to an MAO inhibitor. Treatment is described below. The final option is electroconvulsive therapy (ECT), which is a highly effective, albeit costly, form of treatment for depression.

*Note* that the clinician must wait 2 weeks after discontinuing typical antidepressants before beginning an MAOI, and six weeks after discontinuing fluoxetine before a switch to an MAOI. Failure to do so may result in very serious and potentially life-threatening drug interactions.

## Dysthymia

Dysthymia is a type of mild, chronic depressive disorder characterized by the following symptoms (which are present almost every day over a period of 2+ years):
- Daytime fatigue
- Negative, pessimistic thinking
- Low self-esteem
- Low motivation, loss of enthusiasm
- Decreased capacity for joy

Evidence from a number of recent studies suggests that approximately two-thirds of patients with dysthymia can respond favorably to a trial on anti-depressant

## Figure 10

## SELECTIVE ACTION OF ANTIDEPRESSANT MEDICATIONS[1]

| GENERIC | BRAND | NOREPINEPHRINE NE | SEROTONIN 5-HT | MONOAMINE OXIDASE | DOPAMINE DA |
|---|---|---|---|---|---|
| imipramine | Tofranil | ++ | +++ | 0 | 0 |
| desipramine | Norpramin | +++++ | 0 | 0 | 0 |
| amitriptyline | Elavil | ++ | ++++ | 0 | 0 |
| nortriptyline | Aventyl, Pamelor | +++ | ++ | 0 | 0 |
| protriptyline | Vivactil | ++++ | + | 0 | 0 |
| trimipramine | Surmontil | ++ | ++ | 0 | 0 |
| doxepin | Sinequan, Adapin | +++ | ++ | 0 | 0 |
| maprotiline | Ludiomil | +++++ | 0 | 0 | 0 |
| amoxapine | Asendin | ++++ | ++ | 0 | 0 |
| venlafaxine | Effexor | ++ | +++ | 0 | + |
| desvenlafaxine | Pristiq | ++ | +++ | 0 | + |
| trazodone | Desyrel | 0 | +++++ | 0 | 0 |
| fluoxetine | Prozac | 0 | +++++ | 0 | 0 |
| paroxetine | Paxil | + | +++++ | 0 | 0 |
| sertraline | Zoloft | 0 | +++++ | 0 | 0 |
| bupropion | Wellbutrin[2] | +++ | 0 | 0 | ++ |
| nefazodone | Serzone | + | ++++ | 0 | 0 |
| fluvoxamine | Luvox | 0 | +++++ | 0 | 0 |
| mirtazapine | Remeron | ++ | +++ | 0 | 0 |
| citalopram | Celexa | 0 | +++++ | 0 | 0 |
| escitalopram | Lexapro | 0 | +++++ | 0 | 0 |
| duloxetine | Cymbalta | ++++ | ++++ | 0 | 0 |
| atomoxetine | Strattera | +++++ | 0 | 0 | 0 |
| reboxetine | Vestra | +++++ | 0 | 0 | 0 |
| phenelzine | Nardil[3] | +++ | +++ | +++++ | +++ |
| tranylcypromine | Parnate[3] | +++ | +++ | +++++ | +++ |
| isocarboxazid | Marplan[3] | +++ | +++ | +++++ | +++ |
| selegiline | Emsam | +++ | +++ | +++++ | +++ |

[1]0 = no impact on neurotransmitter; + = minimal impact, +++++ = significant impact.
[2]Atypical antidepressant. Uncertain effects.
[3]MAOIs increase NE, 5-HT, and DA

medications. MAOIs and SSRIs appear to be more effective than tricyclics in treating dysthymia.

## Major Depression with Atypical Symptoms

15–20% of major depressions present with what are referred to as *atypical symptoms,* which include: hypersomnia (excessive sleeping), significant weight gain, carbohydrate craving, and extreme fatigue. It is important to note that this is the most common clinical presentation of depression in patients with bipolar illness. As will be addressed in the next chapter, treatment of bipolar depression with antidepressants alone carries risks of precipitating a shift into mania and/or cycle acceleration. Thus the clinician must always take special note of atypical symptoms and be cautious about treating with antidepressants (see chapter 3 for more details). Atypical symptoms are also the most common presentation seen in seasonal affective disorder.

## Seasonal Affective Disorder (S.A.D.)

Decreased exposure to photic stimulation has been strongly implicated in cases of S.A.D. This is often a factor in people who work at night, live in geographic areas with significant cloud cover and/or pollution, and in northern climes (Northern hemisphere) during winter months. A full discussion of S.A.D. is beyond the scope of this book, but physicians prescribers should be aware of this common clinical condition. Treatment for S.A.D. includes antidepressants (current hypotheses suggest that S.A.D. may be closely tied to serotinergic dysfunction, and thus SSRIs may be medications of choice). Additionally, increased bright light exposure has been shown to be effective (either by use of commercially available light boxes or by encouraging patients to spend a minimum of one hour per day outside . . . of course, without sunglasses). Since many cases of seasonal depression are a manifestation of bipolar disorder, please note that increased bright light exposure can precipitate manias in those with bipolar illness.

For a detailed discussion of S.A.D., please see *Winter Blues* by N.E. Rosenthal, Guilford Press, N.Y. (2006).

## Pre-menstrual Dysphoric Disorder (PMDD)

Approximately 5% of women experience severe mood changes premenstrually. This disorder is characterized by the tremendous regularity of mood symptoms (depression, irritability or anxiety) seen for a few days prior to menstruation. Serotinergic dysregulation has been implicated and treatment with SSRIs is often a successful strategy. Currently, there is some debate whether or not it is necessary to treat PMDD continuously (i.e., all month-long) or on a P.R.N. basis. All other types of depression require chronic treatment, however; some women with PMDD *may* respond to P.R.N. dosing only during the symptomatic time of the month.

## Psychotic Depressions

Psychotic symptoms may be seen in cases of unipolar depression and bipolar disorder, and occur also in the context of postpartum and menopausal depressions. They usually manifest with severe vegetative symptoms, delusions (especially somatic delusions, extreme beliefs regarding worthlessness, and paranoid thinking) and occasionally, auditory hallucinations.

Antidepressants alone or antipsychotics alone are generally ineffective. Almost always the treatment of choice includes a combination of antidepressants and antipsychotics. Electroconvulsive therapy (E.C.T.) may be both necessary and effective in more severe cases. Finally, please keep in mind that these patients are very high risk for suicide. Referral to a psychiatrist and possibly hospitalization are recommended.

## Precautions: Tricyclic Antidepressants

The following patients should either not be treated or treated cautiously with tricyclics: immediate post-myocardial infarction patients, epileptics, patients with narrow-angle glaucoma, and pregnant women. The physician should consult package inserts and the *Physicians' Desk Reference* for more details regarding precautions and contraindications.

## Precautions: Selective Serotonin Reuptake Inhibitors

Drug-drug interactions can sometimes be dangerous. SSRIs should be used *cautiously* with certain medications (Figure 11). Also note that very rare cases of liver toxicity have been reported with the antidepressants nefazodone and atomoxetine.

### *Figure 11*

- MAO Inhibitors—never use with SSRIs (very dangerous/fatal)
- Tricyclic antidepressants (may increase TCA levels)
- Lithium (may increase lithium levels)
- Carbamazepine (may increase carbamazepine levels)
- St. John's Wort (may be dangerous)

*Note:* This list is not exhaustive, but includes common drug-drug interactions

## Precautions: Watch for Bipolar Disorder

Patients with a personal or family history of bipolar disorder often present with depressive symptoms. They may or may not reveal a history of mania. Caution should be exercised in prescribing since all antidepressants can precipitate a shift from depression into mania. It is always advisable to ask the patient (and family members) if there has been a family history of bipolar illness (see Chapter 3) or if any of the following symptoms of possible hypomania have been present for more than one or two days:

- Decreased need for sleep, but without daytime fatigue
- Rapid, pressured speech
- High levels of energy
- Intense irritability
- Racing thoughts

In addition, any of the following may suggest the depressive phase of bipolar disorder: a history of relatively brief major depressions (less than 3 months), a history of a first-onset major depression prior to age 18; psychotic symptoms (e.g. delusions); unsuccessful past treatments with antidepressants (despite adequate trials) or a positive response lasting only a month or two, with a return of depressive symptoms; clear seasonal patterns to depressions (i.e. history of depressions occurring in the winter); and/or the presence of atypical symptoms (as described on page 15).

If a patient presents with any of these characteristics, they should be considered bipolar until proven otherwise.

## MAO Inhibitors

Three commonly used MAOIs (phenelzine, isocarboxazid, selegiline and tranylcypromine) have been shown to be as effective as tricyclics in a number of studies. However, shortly after their introduction into the United States in the 1950s there were reports of severe reactions in some patients, which resulted in great concern in the medical community. The drugs interact with certain medications (sympathomimetic amines) and with certain foods (containing tyramine, a natural byproduct of bacterial fermentation processes, found in many cheeses, some wines and beers, and foods such as chopped liver, broad beans, chocolate, snails, etc.). (See Appendix B.) The interaction resulted in a severe hypertensive crisis, which for a number of patients was fatal. So for many years these medications were abandoned because doctors viewed them as unsafe. However, especially in Europe, doctors recognized that these drugs had clinical utility and could be safely used if certain dietary restrictions were followed. Additionally, the MAOI, Emsam (available in a transdermal patch) if given at a dose of 6 mg per day may not require dietary restrictions (such restrictions however may be necessary at doses of 9-12 mg).

MAOIs should be considered as a third or fourth-line treatment choice, should other antidepressants fail. Additionally, some studies indicate that MAOIs may be the drug of choice for some types of affective disorders including atypical depressions presenting primarily with anxiety and phobic symptoms, masked depression (e.g., hypochondriasis), highly treatment resistant depressions and dysthymia.

Otherwise, guidelines for treatment and clinical response are similar to those previously described for typical antidepressants. The one exception is the important dietary/medication restrictions that must be observed (see Appendix B, patient handout for specific restrictions).

## Notes on Over-the-Counter Products

Several over-the-counter products have been shown to have efficacy in treating depression. Please see chapter 7.

## Books to Recommend to Patients

1. Preston, J. and Kirk, M. (2011) *Depression 101*. New Harbinger Publishers, Oakland, CA.
2. Jefferson, J. and Greist, J.H. (1999). *Depression and Antidepressants: A Guide*, Madison Institute of Medicine, Madison, Wisconsin.

# Chapter 3  Bipolar Illness

## DIAGNOSIS

## Major Clinical Features and Differential Diagnosis

The diagnosis of a bipolar disorder is based on two sources of data: the current clinical picture (depression or mania) and a clear history of both manic and depressive episodes. The depressive episodes may range from minor to major depressive syndromes as outlined in Chapter 2. Manic episodes typically are described as either full blown (Figure 14) or less intense manic episodes, referred to as hypomania.

It is important to rule out medical causes of bipolar illness. (See Figures 1 and 2 in Chapter 2 and Figures 12 and 13.)

*Figure 12*

### COMMON DISORDERS THAT MAY CAUSE MANIA

- Brain tumors
- CNS syphilis
- Delirium (due to various causes)
- Encephalitis
- Influenza
- Metabolic changes associated with hemodialysis
- Metastatic squamous adenocarcinoma
- Multiple sclerosis
- Q fever

*Figure 13*

### DRUGS THAT MAY CAUSE MANIA

- amphetamines
- bromides
- cocaine
- antidepressants
- isoniazid
- procarbazine
- steroids
- stimulants

Several classification schemes for bipolar disorders have been proposed by various authors. The three most clinically useful classifications are outlined below:

## A. BIPOLAR I vs. BIPOLAR II

1. *Bipolar I*   This disorder fits the more classic description of bipolar illness with clearly recognized episodes of depression and mania.

2. *Bipolar II*   This disorder presents with obvious episodes of depression; but the manic phases of the illness are often brief, much less intense, unrecognized, and thus not reported by the patient. If you inquire about manic episodes, the patient will often give the impression that none have occurred. The best ways to diagnose such conditions are either to witness a hypomanic episode (see Figure 14) clinically or to carefully inquire about the history. In particular, if hypomanic episodes are suspected, the most important question to ask is, "Have you ever had a period of time when you didn't need as much sleep?" A decreased need for sleep and a lack of daytime fatigue are red flags for hypomania. Typical hypomanic episodes only last 1–4 days. Many cases of apparent treatment-resistant depression may turn out to be bipolar II (they always present with depressive symptoms and many times do not respond well to treatments with antidepressants). Additionally, treatment with antidepressants alone can cause a shift into hypomania. Often it is very helpful to obtain information from a spouse or close relative; family members often clearly can identify a history of past hypomanias where patients cannot.

## B. TYPICAL BIPOLAR vs. RAPID CYCLING BIPOLAR DISORDERS

In the more typical bipolar patient, depressive and manic episodes last for several weeks to several months, often with periods of normal mood occurring between periods of depression and mania. When there are two or more episodes of *both* depression and mania (e.g., depression-mania-depression-mania) within a year, this is referred to as "rapid cycling." Sometimes rapid cyclers (RC) can dramatically switch moods from week to week or even day to day. RC can best be seen as periods of exacerbation of bipolar disorder that are episodic (e.g. those who experience RC may do so for six months or a year, and then return to more typical episodes of mania and depression). Substance abuse or treatment with antidepressants are common factors in provoking RC and should always be evaluated in those with RC symptomatology.

## C. DYSPHORIC MANIA (or MIXED MANIA)

This is a diagnostic term which describes patients that have concurrent manic and depressive symptoms (e.g., increased activity or agitation, pressured speech, suicidal ideas, and feelings of worthlessness) (see Figure 14).

The subclassifications of Bipolar I and Bipolar II, typical vs. rapid cycling, and dysphoric mania are important because they have different treatment implications.

## Target Symptoms

The target symptoms vary depending on the current phase of the illness. Major depressive symptoms are listed in Chapter 2 (Figures 3 and 4). Manic episodes are identified by the following clinical features (see Figure 14).

## MEDICATIONS USED TO TREAT BIPOLAR ILLNESS

## When Do You Prescribe Medications?

Treatment of bipolar disorders has two goals. The first goal is the reduction of current symptoms, and the second is the prevention of relapse. Bipolar disorders are invariably recurring and thus prophylactic treatment is warranted. Although prevention of episode recurrence is a goal, in reality only about one in five will, with appropriate treatment, avoid subsequent episodes. The more common outcome is that appropriate treatment can significantly reduce the number and frequency of episodes. Unfortunately, even more common is that patients are non-compliant with medication treatment (typically owing to side effects) and the result is ongoing recurrences. Strong evidence indicates that failure to continue treatment can lead (and often does) not only to relapse, but to a progressively worsening condition. Subsequent episodes tend to become more and more severe and can, at times, become treatment refractory.

## Choosing Medication

An important medication used to treat this disorder is lithium (has the best track record providing long-term mood stabilization). Also it is important to note that several large-scale studies have shown that patients treated with lithium show a significant decrease in suicides (a 7-fold reduction in suicide rates). Thus although treatment with lithium can be challenging owing to the need for numerous blood tests and other types of laboratory monitoring, this drug continues to play an important role in the treatment of bipolar disorder. A number of other drugs have been found to be effective as adjuncts or alternatives to lithium. We will describe standard treatment with lithium and then comment on the role of other medications.

Lithium has two primary effects: It is used to treat acute mood episodes (i.e. it is used to treat acute manic and depressive episodes), and in many instances it can prevent relapse (or at least lessen the intensity of subsequent episodes) if treatment is on an ongoing basis. Lithium seems to be somewhat more effective in preventing relapse of mania rather than depression.

## Prescribing Treatment

The treatment of bipolar disorders can be quite complex. Generally a referral to a specialist is recommended, although recently there has been pressure on primary care physicians to treat this disorder.

## Figure 14

## SYMPTOMS OF MANIA[1]

- A pronounced and persistent mood of euphoria (elevated or expansive mood) or irritability and at least three of the following:
- Grandiosity or elevated self-esteem
- Decreased need for sleep
- Rapid, pressured speech (Often these people are hard, if not impossible, to interrupt.)
- Racing thoughts
- Distractibility
- Increased activity or psychomotor agitation
- Behavior that reflects expansiveness (lacking restraint in emotional expression) and poor judgment, such as increased sexual promiscuity, gambling, buying sprees, giving away money, etc.

## SYMPTOMS OF DYSPHORIC MANIA

- Marked irritability
- Severe agitation or anxiety
- Pessimism and unrelenting worry and despair
- Significant suicide risk
- Decreased need for sleep

## SYMPTOMS OF HYPOMANIA

- Increased energy and mental productivity
- Decreased need for sleep
- Talkative
- Elated, mildly grandiose
- Irritability

---

[1]See Questions 13–16 on the History and Personal Data Questionnaire (Appendix A.).

*If the presenting phase is a manic episode.* Often, especially if the patient is quite agitated, out of control or psychotic, the initial plan is to begin treatment with *both* an anti-manic agent and an antipsychotic medication (e.g., olanzapine). The antipsychotics seem to improve behavioral control more rapidly. With most standard anti-manic medications, the patient may require 10 days to show a clinical response. Alternatively, high potency benzodiazepines can be used in place of antipsychotics (e.g., clonazepam or lorazepam).

## Figure 15

## DECISION TREE FOR TREATMENT OF BIPOLAR DISORDERS

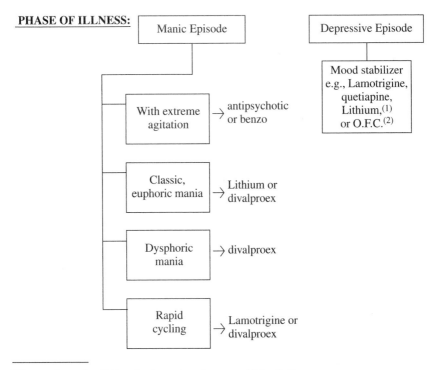

[1]To treat depression, lithium levels must reach or exceed 0.8 mEq/L.
[2]OFC: olanzapine-fluoxetine combination (Symbyax)

Treatment with lithium is initiated after necessary lab tests are conducted (see Figure 16). Generally the starting dose is 600 or 900 mg./day given in divided doses. The therapeutic range and toxic range of lithium are very close to one another. Thus it is necessary to gradually increase the dose while carefully monitoring blood levels. Most patients must reach a level between 1.0 and 1.2 mEq/L. Not infrequently the level may need to be higher to obtain symptomatic improvement (1.2 to 1.5), but on these higher levels, side effects are more common and compliance is poorer. On occasion, patients may need and tolerate blood levels up to 2.0 mEq/L. However, there is increased risk of toxicity at such doses. Generally, daily doses range from 1200-3000 mg. Once mood is adequately stabilized, the dose can be lowered somewhat (0.8 mEq/L blood level for Bipolar I or 0.6 mEq/L for Bipolar II) for maintenance treatment.

Major side effects include nausea, diarrhea, vomiting, fine hand tremor, sedation, muscular weakness, polyuria, polydypsia, edema, weight gain and a dry mouth. Adverse effects from chronic use may include leukocytosis (reversible upon discontinuation of lithium), hypothyroidism and goiter, acne, psoriasis, teratogenesis (first trimester, although the risk is very low), nephrogenic diabetes insipidus (reversible), and, rarely, kidney damage.

Signs of toxicity include lethargy, ataxia, slurred speech, tinnitus, severe nausea/vomiting, tremor, arrhythmias, hypotension, seizures, shock, delirium, coma, and even death. Since the toxic range is near to the therapeutic range, blood levels and adverse effects must be monitored closely. In addition, a number of other clinical lab tests should be conducted at the beginning of treatment and periodically thereafter (see Figure 16).

*Figure 16*

**CLINICAL LAB TESTS FOR PATIENTS TAKING LITHIUM**

- NA (Sodium)
- Ca (Calcium)
- P (Phosphorus)
- EKG

- Creatinine
- Urinalysis
- Complete CBC
- Thyroid battery (with TSH)

Other antimanic agents can be used alone or in combination with lithium. These include: mood-stabilizing anticonvulsants: divalproex, carbamazepine, oxcarbazepine, or antipsychotics (all antipsychotics have potent antimanic effects). Most anticonvulsants have significant side effects and some are known teratogens. Common side effects include: nausea, fine hand tremor, sedation, weight gain (all except topiramate), rash, menstrual irregularities (please see PDR or package inserts for specific adverse effects associated with each of the anticonvulsant mood stabilizers). Generally the newer antipsychotics are used; e.g. olanzapine, risperidone, paliperidone, ziprasidone, quetiapine, or aripiprazole (see chapter 5 for more details on antipsychotic medications).

*If the presenting phase is a depressive episode.* Antidepressants alone in the treatment of bipolar depression may cause significant problems, by provoking a rapid shift into mania (and also may increase the subsequent frequency of episodes; i.e. causing cycle acceleration). Antidepressants as a monotherapy are not advised. Thus, typically the treatment of choice is to use one of the four following medications: lamotrigine, olanzapine-fluoxetine combination (OFC, brand name: Symbyax), quetiapine or lithium. Should this strategy fail, often a combination of two or more of these medications is effective. *Medication combinations are almost always necessary*: 90% of successfully treated bipolar patients require polypharmacy (e.g. lithium and quetiapine).

| NAMES | | Daily | Serum[1] |
|-------|------|-------|-------|
| Generic | Brand | Dosage Range | Level |
| carbamazepine | Tegretol | 600–1600 | 4–10+ |
| oxcarbazepine | Trileptal | 1200–2400 | (2) |
| divalproex | Depakote | 750–1500 | 50–100 |
| lamotrigine | Lamictal | 200–500 | (2) |

1. Serum levels are necessary for some anticonvulsants during the beginning stages of treatment and several times per year after or when there are emergent side effects or dosage increases.
2. Serum monitoring may not be necessary

## *Figure 17*

## SPECIALIZED TREATMENTS FOR SUBTYPES
## OF BIPOLAR DISORDERS

| SUBTYPE | MEDICATION ALTERNATIVES |
|---|---|
| Bipolar II | Quetiapine or O.F.C. |
| Rapid Cyclers | Lamotrigine |
| Dysphoric Mania | Divalproex |

For details on alternative treatment approaches see the following:

*Practice Guidelines for Treatment of Patients with Bi-Polar Disorder.* Hirschfeld, RMA, et al. (2002) Practice Guidelines for the treatment of patients with bipolar disorder (revision). *American Journal of Psychiatry,* 159: 1–50.

## Common Treatment Errors to Avoid

- Lithium: very toxic thus warrants close monitoring (especially in suicidal patients. *Note:* Suicides occur frequently not only in depressed but also manic patients). Acute dehydration can also result in toxic lithium levels.
- Poor compliance
- Discontinuation: *Note:* Bipolar patients need life-long treatment to avoid relapse. Patient or physician-initiated discontinuation can and does result in frequent relapses. And, subsequent episodes often are more severe and may become treatment-resistant. If discontinuation must occur, it is strongly recommended that it be done gradually (e.g., over a period of 6 weeks).

# KEY POINTS TO COMMUNICATE TO PATIENTS

1. Lithium and other bipolar drugs are medications that treat your current emotional problem and will also be helpful in preventing relapse. So it will be important to continue with treatment after the current episode is resolved.

2. Since the therapeutic and toxic dosage ranges (lithium) are so close, we must monitor your blood level closely. Some anticonvulsant mood stabilizers also must have periodic monitoring. This will be done more frequently at first and every several months thereafter. Never increase your dose without first consulting with your physician.

3. Lithium and other bipolar medications are not addictive.

4. Many side effects can be reduced/minimized by taking divided doses or may subside as treatment progresses.

5. Bipolar disorders often run in families. Any relatives who have pronounced mood swings should be alerted to the possibility of a treatable condition and the need for professional evaluation. (The yield on this maneuver is high, since medical awareness of bipolar disorder is still low, especially with milder forms, and family history is impressively often positive for this disorder.)

6. You and your family need to be aware that this is a biological disorder, not a moral defect or a character flaw. When severe, you may not always be able to control your behavior, necessitating that practical steps be taken to protect all concerned from poor judgment during episodes.

7. Many self-help groups have been developed to provide support for bipolar patients and their families. In this community, the local self-help group is ____ , and you can find out more information by calling ____ .

8. Anticonvulsant mood stabilizers can cause birth defects so if you become pregnant or plan a pregnancy please contact your prescriber immediately.

9. Lifestyle management is especially important in maintaining stability. This cannot be overemphasized; without this critical ingredient, medication treatments often fail. Lifestyle management includes:

   - Maintaining regular bedtimes and times for awakening
   - Avoid sleep deprivation (even one night can be problematic)
   - Avoid shift work
   - Attempt to keep the amount of bright (sunlight) exposure stable throughout the year (note: decreased light exposure in the winter often provokes bipolar depression while excessive sunlight exposure in the summer often ignites mania).
   - Avoid the use of alcohol and any illicit drug use
   - Avoid substances that interfere with sleep: caffeine, alcohol, minor tranquilizers, decongestants, etc.
   - If possible avoid or limit travel across time zones.

## Books to Recommend to Patients

1. Jamison, K. R. (1997). *Unquiet Mind,* Random House, New York.

2. Fast, J. and Preston, J. (2004) *Loving Someone with Bipolar Disorder.* New Harbinger Publications, Oakland, CA.

3. Fast, J. and Preston, J. (2006) *Taking Charge of Bipolar Disorder.* Warner Wellness Books. New York.

4. White, R. and Preston, J. (2010) *Bipolar Disorder 101.* New Harbinger Publications, Oakland, CA.

# Chapter 4   Anxiety Disorders

## DIAGNOSIS

### Major Clinical Features and Differential Diagnosis

Six different anxiety disorders are seen in clinical practice.[1] An accurate diagnosis is important as the treatments vary. There is no one treatment appropriate for all anxiety disorders. It is important to distinguish between the following: (1) generalized anxiety disorder (G.A.D.), (2) stress-related anxiety, (3) panic disorder, (4) social phobias, (5) medical illnesses presenting with anxiety symptoms, and (6) anxiety symptoms as a part of a primary mental disorder (e.g., depression, schizophrenia).

Before outlining the main features of each disorder, it is necessary to define two terms: panic attacks and anxiety symptoms. Panic attacks are very brief but extremely intense surges of anxiety. The major differences between a panic attack and more generalized anxiety symptoms are differences in the onset, duration, and intensity. Panic attacks often "come out of the blue" (i.e., not necessarily provoked by stress), they come on suddenly (the full attack reaching its peak in from one-to-ten minutes), are *extremely* intense, last from 1–30 minutes, and then subside. The patient feels as if he will actually die or go crazy. We are not talking about uneasiness; we are talking about full-blown panic. The person may continue to feel nervous or upset for several hours, but the attack itself lasts only a matter of minutes. If a patient says, "I've had a continuous panic attack for the past three days," he may be having intense anxiety symptoms, but not a true panic attack. In other anxiety disorders, anxiety symptoms can be very unpleasant, but are much less intense; they also can be prolonged or generalized (i.e., present most of the day and last from days to years). The distinction between "symptoms" and "attacks" is very important when it comes to treatment. Please refer to Figure 18.

The six anxiety syndromes can be distinguished by the following characteristics:

1. *Generalized Anxiety Disorder.* The key here is *long-term,* low level, fairly continuous anxiety. Patients with this disorder *may* have no specific current life stressors. To them, daily living provokes anxiety. Such people are chronic

---

[1]Note: Obsessive-Compulsive disorder and Post-traumatic stress disorder are discussed in Chapter 6.

*Figure 18*

## SYMPTOMS OF ANXIETY

- Trembling, feeling shaky, restlessness, muscle tension
- Shortness of breath, smothering sensation
- Tachycardia (rapid heartbeat)
- Sweating and cold hands and feet
- Lightheadedness and dizziness
- Paresthesias (tingling of the skin)
- Diarrhea and/or frequent urination
- Feelings of unreality (derealization)
- Initial insomnia (difficulty falling asleep)
- Impaired attention and concentration
- Nervousness, edginess, or tension

worriers, always "what-if-ing" (e.g., "What if I get fired?" "What if my check bounces?" "What if my wife leaves me?").

2. *Stress-related Anxiety.* The patient with this disorder typically functions well. However, the anxiety symptoms have recently emerged in the face of major life stresses (e.g., a serious family illness, a marital separation, etc.).

3. *Panic Disorder.* This is characterized by repeated episodes of full-blown panic, as described in the discussion of panic attacks. Often phobias will also develop.

4. *Social Anxiety.* Anxiety is experienced only when the person is in social/interpersonal settings, e.g., public speaking, asking someone out for a date, social gatherings.

5. *Medical Illnesses, and Medications Presenting with Anxiety Symptoms.* Certain diseases/conditions can at times result in biochemical changes that produce anxiety symptoms. If someone complains of nervousness or anxiety, it should never be assumed that it is simply an emotional disorder until medical causes have been ruled out (Figure 19). Likewise, a number of medications and over-the-counter products can cause pronounced anxiety symptoms (Figure 20).

6. *Anxiety as a Part of a Primary Mental Disorder.* Anxiety frequently accompanies many mental disorders (e.g., depression, schizophrenia, organic brain syndromes, substance abuse).

*Figure 19*

## COMMON DISORDERS THAT MAY CAUSE ANXIETY

- Adrenal tumor
- Alcoholism
- Angina pectoris
- Cardiac arrhythmia
- CNS degenerative diseases
- Cushing's disease
- Coronary insufficiency
- Delirium[1]

- Hypoglycemia
- Hyperthyroidism
- Meniere's disease (early stages)
- Mitral valve prolapse[2]
- Parathyroid disease
- Partial-complex seizures
- Post-concussion syndrome
- Premenstrual syndrome

---

[1]Delirium can occur as a result of many toxic/metabolic conditions and often produces anxiety and agitation.
[2]The mitral valve prolapse probably does not cause anxiety, but it has been found that MVP and anxiety disorders often coexist. This may be due to some underlying common genetic factor.

*Figure 20*

## DRUGS THAT MAY CAUSE ANXIETY

- Amphetamines
- Appetite suppressants
- Asthma medications
- Caffeine
- CNS depressants (withdrawal)
- Cocaine
- Nasal decongestants
- Steroids
- Stimulants

# ANTIANXIETY MEDICATION* TREATMENT

## When Do You Prescribe Antianxiety Medications?

Treatment differs depending on the diagnosis, so each disorder will be addressed separately.

1. *Generalized Anxiety Disorder (G.A.D.).* Many physicians have tried to treat this disorder with benzodiazepines. This presents two problems: (1) Benzodiazepines

---

*Also referred to as minor tranquilizers, anxiolytics, and benzodiazepines. These terms will be used interchangeably.

can cause depression in some individuals, (2) patients can develop tolerance/dependence problems with chronic benzodiazepine use. Many clinicians think that G.A.D. is primarily a psychological (not biological) disorder and recommend psychotherapy. However, SSRIs, venlafaxine and buspirone hydrochloride, have been shown to be effective in treating G.A.D. An added feature of these medications is that patients do not develop dependence or tolerance.

2. *Stress-related anxiety.* Minor tranquilizers are very helpful in reducing anxiety symptoms (especially insomnia and restlessness) which accompany acute situational stress. The most important issue to consider is whether or not the stress is acute and likely to be of short duration. Antianxiety medications should only be used for a period of 1–4 weeks. If it is clear that this is just one in a series of chronic life crises, it is probably best not to prescribe benzodiazepines.

3. *Panic disorder.* One isolated panic attack is generally insufficient evidence of true panic disorder. However, four or more true attacks within a period of one month suggest panic disorder. Look for spontaneous attacks (most "come out of the blue") and episodes that last a matter of minutes (not hours or days). Many patients with other types of disorders say they have panic attacks but on close inspection, many do not.

4. *Social phobias.* Generally, social phobias are not treated medically but with psychotherapy and behavioral approaches. In some cases beta blockers, MAO inhibitors, venlafaxine or SSRIs have been helpful.

5. *Medical illnesses/medications causing anxiety symptoms.* In almost all instances, the treatment of choice is to treat the primary medical illness or to discontinue the offending drug. Be cautious in stopping certain drugs; for instance, if a patient stops drinking coffee abruptly, he may have significant withdrawal symptoms which mimic anxiety. Such drugs must be gradually withdrawn.

6. *Anxiety symptoms as a part of another primary mental disorder.* Treat the primary disorder. Minor tranquilizers are usually not indicated.

## Choosing a Medication

Antianxiety medications fall into five groups (see Figure 21). The primary choice of medication is based on the diagnosis. Secondarily, one should consider certain problematic side effects such as sedation and rapidity of absorption (rapid absorption may be associated with a euphoric "rush").

## Prescribing Treatment

1. *Generalized Anxiety Disorder.* There are several options, including buspirone. Unlike the benzodiazepines, buspirone is slow acting. It often requires 2–6 weeks

of treatment before symptomatic improvement. The major problem encountered with this medication is premature discontinuation by the patient. Patients often expect quick results from medications. It is important to educate the patient about onset of action. Buspirone can be effective in treating many symptoms of G.A.D., but it does not seem to decrease panic attacks. Buspirone must be taken every day; it is not a medication that is taken only when the patient feels anxious. SSRIs or venlafaxine may also be beneficial in treating G.A.D. Again, treatment requires 2–6 weeks before signs of symptomatic improvement emerge. If patients fail to respond to buspirone, venlafaxine, or SSRIs, if symptoms are severe, and if there is no history of alcohol or other substance abuse, benzodiazepines can be used to treat G.A.D.

2. *Stress-Related Anxiety.* All benzodiazepines are effective in treating acute stress-induced anxiety. (See Figure 21). The most important considerations in choosing a medication have to do with side effects and medication half life. The most common side effect is sedation. Intense restlessness or agitation may require a more sedating drug; however, in most instances it is better to use low sedation benzodiazepines to reduce daytime anxiety. Of course many anxious patients will present with a sleep disturbance. Insomnia will be addressed below. A second side effect is the so-called euphoric "rush" secondary to the peak in blood level of medication. Such a peak creates a good deal of sedation and can be useful if the goal is to induce sleep, but the euphoric experience can lead to abuse. In addiction-prone individuals it is best to choose a drug that avoids or minimizes this effect. Finally the half life of a medication is an important variable when it comes to discontinuing the drug (see below). Those medications listed that have a shorter half life may need to be discontinued *very* gradually so as to avoid withdrawal symptoms.

Dosage ranges vary widely as seen in Figure 21. However, a typical starting dose of lorazepam, for instance, is 0.5 mg. b.i.d. or t.i.d. Such a dose should be increased every three days as needed until a final range of 2–6 mg./day is achieved. The goal is to provide some symptomatic relief over a period of from 1–4 weeks. Should a person still experience significant anxiety after this period of time, a reassessment of the diagnosis and referral to a psychotherapist is in order.

It has long been held that long-term use of benzodiazepines is contraindicated. Although this is often true, it is not always the case. Investigations into chronic benzodiazepine use have shed new light on this clinical practice. At times patients will continue to derive benefit from long-term treatment with benzodiazepines. The key is to monitor closely for signs of increasing dosage, especially as the patient may be increasing dosage without medical advice. If in doubt, don't hesitate to get a blood level and to share your concerns openly with the patient. Addiction to benzodiazepines that arise in the course of the treatment of anxiety should be treated for what it is: an occasional and serious side effect. *Always* discontinue benzodiazepines gradually (e.g., if the patient takes 1.5 mg. of alprazolam, q.d., then each week the daily dose should be reduced by 0.25 mg. This slow taper is especially important with short half-life benzodiazepines).

## Figure 21

## ANTIANXIETY MEDICATIONS

| Disorder | Medication Generic | Medication Brand | Usual Daily Dosage Range | Rapidity of Absorption | ½ Life (Hours) |
|---|---|---|---|---|---|
| 1. G.A.D. | buspirone SSRIs[1] | BuSpar | 5–40 mg. | + | 2–8 |
| 2. Stress-Related Anxiety | diazepam | Valium | 5–40 mg. | +++++ | 20–50 |
| | chlordiazepoxide | Librium | 15–100 mg. | +++ | 5–30 |
| | oxazepam | Serax | 30–120 mg. | ++ | 5–20 |
| | clorazepate | Tranxene | 15–60 mg. | ++++ | 30–100 |
| | lorazepam | Ativan | 2–6 mg. | +++ | 10–15 |
| | prazepam | Centrax | 20–60 mg. | + | 30–100 |
| | alprazolam | Xanax | .25–4 mg. | +++ | 6–20 |
| | clonazepam | Klonopin | .5–4 mg. | + | 80 |
| 3. Panic Disorder | alprazolam | Xanax | .25–.8 mg. | +++ | 6–20 |
| | lorazepam | Ativan | 2–6 mg. | +++ | 10–15 |
| | clonazepam antidepressants[1] MAO Inhibitors[1] | Klonopin | .5–4 mg. | + | 80 |
| 4. Social Phobia | propranolol SSRIs[1] venlafaxine[1] MAO Inhibitors[1] | Inderal | 20–80mg. | | |
| 5. Stress-Related Initial Insomnia[2] | flurazepam | Dalmane | 15–30 mg. | +++++ | 40–250[3] |
| | temazepam | Restoril | 15–30 mg. | +++++ | 10–20 |
| | triazolam | Halcion | .25–.5 mg. | +++++ | 2–3 |
| | quazepam | Doral | 7.5–15 mg. | +++++ | 39 |
| | zolpidem | Ambien | 5–10 mg. | ++++ | 2–3 |
| | estazolam | Prosom | 2–4 mg. | +++++ | 10–24 |
| | zaleplon | Sonata | 5–10 mg. | +++++ | 1–2 |
| | eszopiclone[4] | Lunesta | 1–3 mg. | +++++ | 6 |
| | ramelteon[4] | Rozerem | 8 mg. | +++++ | 1–3 |

[1]See Chapter 2, Figure 5.
[2]Initial insomnia: difficulty falling asleep.
[3]Active metabolite (norflurazepam)
[4]non habit-forming

3. *Stress-Induced Insomnia.* Benzodiazepine sedative-hypnotics can be a safe and effective treatment for transient initial insomnia. (Recall that middle insomnia and early morning awakening are more indicative of depression and therefore should not be treated with benzodiazepines). Again, in most cases treatment is initiated only if the insomnia is precipitated by recent environ-

mental stress and is not a chronic problem. Chronic insomnia is extremely hard to treat. Note that the drug zolpidem tartrate is not a benzodiazepine and studies to date show that dependence is less likely with this medication. For this reason, it may be a safe alternative in individuals with a substance abuse history. Typical dosages for the various sedatives are listed in Figure 21. Another popular drug of choice that has no addiction potential is the sedating antidepressant trazodone (dosing: 25–100 mg. qhs).

4. *Panic Disorder.* The treatment of panic disorder has two discrete phases.

*Phase One:* Eliminate or reduce the frequency or intensity of the panic attacks with antipanic drugs. There are three main groups of antipanic drugs. Let's discuss the pros and cons of each.

a. High potency benzodiazepines and like compounds (e.g., alprazolam, lorazepam, and clonazepam)

*Pros.* Very effective. It works quickly. It also reduces anticipatory anxiety.

*Cons.* Although some patients respond to low doses (0.25 mg t.i.d.), most require much larger doses (3–8 mg/day for alprazolam, 2–4 mg/day for clonazepam), and at these higher doses, sedation is a very common problem. Note: effective panic control only occurs when patients take medications on a regular 24-hour-a-day basis (i.e., *not* P.R.N.). With prolonged use, dependence will develop. *Very* gradual discontinuation is required to avoid withdrawal symptoms.

b. Antidepressants: tricyclics, selective serotonin re-uptake inhibitors (SSRIs), venlafaxine, mirtazapine.

*Pros.* Effective in reducing attacks. Can treat concurrent depression. Can be used for prolonged periods of time without risk of tolerance/dependence.

*Cons.* Side effects (see Chapter 2) and delayed onset of action (2–4 weeks before symptomatic improvement). Treat in the same way and same dosage levels as you would use to treat depression. Many patients experience an initial increase in panic attacks; these are usually managed well with short term use (during the first month of treatment) of a benzodiazepine, as necessary. (Note: Bupropion is one antidepressant that apparently is not effective in treating panic attacks.)

c. MAO Inhibitors

*Pros.* Very effective. Can treat concurrent depression. Can be used for prolonged periods of time without risk of tolerance/dependence.

*Cons.* Delayed onset of action (2–4 weeks) and medication/dietary restrictions as outlined in Chapter 2. As with typical antidepressants, treat as you would treat depression.

*Phase Two.* Patients not only have the attacks, but develop significant anticipatory anxiety, phobias, and avoidance (a strong urge to avoid situations in which they have experienced prior panic attacks, e.g., to avoid crowded stores or driving on freeways). These problems frequently do not spontaneously remit when the panic attacks are eliminated. People continue to have intense worries that "It could happen again." Phase two involves gradual reexposure to feared situations. So, for instance, if a person is afraid of having an attack at the grocery store, he must gradually approach the feared situation. Only by repeated exposure to the situation and by a series of experiences without panic will the patient's anticipatory anxiety and avoidance diminish. The keys to successful graded reexposure are (1) to first effectively control or reduce attacks with medication and then (2) to have the patient very gradually face the phobic situation. To be effective, exposures should last for at least 60 minutes.

The duration of the underlying biochemical dysfunction is quite variable. Some people may be treated medically for six months and gradually withdrawn from medication. Others may need years of continued treatment. Like depression, the strategy with any of the antipanic drugs is to achieve symptomatic relief and then continue to treat for at least 6 months. At that point, a medication-reduction trial may be initiated. If necessary, treatment can be resumed if panic symptoms reemerge.

5. *Social Anxiety.* In most cases psychotherapy is the treatment of choice. Psychotropic medications have been used, however, in two types of social phobia. Some social phobics are extremely sensitive to rejection and this is why they are fearful of social interactions. Clinical data indicate that these patients may benefit from MAO inhibitors, venlafaxine, or SSRIs. A second type of phobia, stage fright/public speaking phobia, has been successfully treated by beta blockers such as propanolol (usually 20–40 mg., 1 hour prior to performing). Beta blockers do not eliminate the centrally mediated, subjective sense of anxiety, but do quite effectively reduce many peripheral somatic symptoms of anxiety, e.g., tachycardia, trembling.

## Common Treatment Errors to Avoid

- As noted in Chapter 2, SSRIs frequently present with increased anxiety as a side effect during the first few weeks of treatment. This is *very* problematic in the treatment of anxiety disorders and a major cause of patient-initiated discontinuation. As mentioned in Chapter 2, it is common practice to co-administer an SSRI and a minor tranquilizer during the first month of treatment (e.g., 0.25–0.5 mg lorazepam, bid or tid). Generally, SSRIs begin to significantly reduce anxiety by week four of treatment, and at this time the tranquilizer can be discontinued.
- Prescribing benzodiazepines to a patient with a personal or family history of substance abuse (high risk of abusing the benzodiazepine). Watch for patient requests for higher and higher doses. In those with a history of or high risk for substance abuse there are four commonly used, non-habit-forming alternatives: trazodone (50–75 mg qhs for sleep), buspirone for generalized anxiety disorder, mirtazapine (7.5–15 mg qhs for sleep), hydroxyzine: Vistaril, Atarax, and gabapentin (300–2400 mg qd) for generalized or stress-related anxiety.

- "Cold turkey" discontinuation or rapid taper of benzodiazepines (can result in significant withdrawal symptoms. 1–3 month gradual taper advised).
- Misdiagnosis: failure to recognize depression or an emerging psychotic illness and treating with benzodiazepines (can worsen depression and fail to treat psychosis).
- Over-sedation with benzodiazepines in the treatment of day-time anxiety.
- Benzodiazepines in treating elderly patients can cause cognitive impairment and contribute to unsteady gait and falls. Use with caution.
- Patients with anxiety disorders should consume *no* caffeine and partial responses or break-through symptoms are often due to unreported caffeine use.

## *IN EVERY CASE, REMEMBER*

Some degree of stress and anxiety is a common part of normal, daily living. Medication treatment should only be initiated if symptoms are significantly intense and severely interfere with normal functioning.

When you prescribe any kind of medication to control anxiety, it is essential to discuss the following key points with the patient:

# KEY POINTS TO COMMUNICATE TO PATIENTS

*All patients suffering from anxiety disorders:* Caffeine use should be zero and regular exercise is a very high yield intervention.

*Generalized Anxiety Disorder*
1. If buspirone, venlafaxine, or SSRIs are prescribed, you should expect that it will take from 2–6 weeks to notice symptomatic improvement. Daily doses are required. This is not a medication that you take only as needed.
2. Often medication treatment is not enough, and psychotherapy, stress management, relaxation training, regular exercise, and biofeedback are helpful adjuncts to medical treatment.

*Stress-Related Anxiety*
1. The following analogy is helpful. Pain killers can reduce suffering when you have a toothache, but at some point you must fix or pull the tooth. Likewise, minor tranquilizers do not cure people, but they temporarily reduce suffering. You must do something to alter the basic source of stress if lasting recovery is to be achieved. Minor tranquilizers are only for short-term use.
2. Do not abruptly discontinue minor tranquilizers, especially if they have been taken daily for several weeks. Cold-turkey discontinuation can result in withdrawal syndromes (many withdrawal symptoms are almost identical to symptoms of anxiety).
3. Do not drink any kind of alcohol if you are taking a minor tranquilizer.

*Figure 22*

# DECISION TREE FOR DIAGNOSIS AND TREATMENT OF ANXIETY

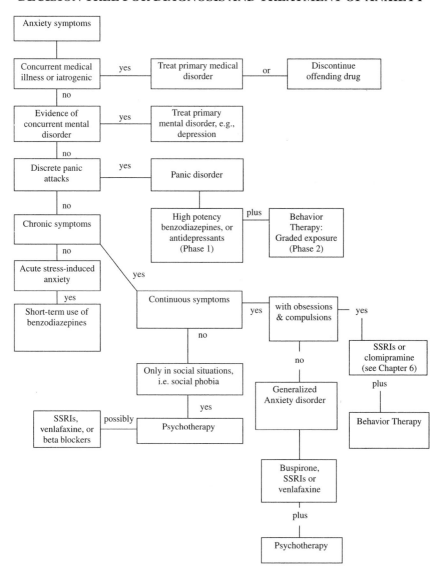

*Panic Disorder*

1. There is strong evidence that panic disorder is a biochemical dysfunction, not a psychological disorder. It can often be very successfully treated with medications.
2. Medication must be taken each day. The treatment is prophylactic and not a medication that you only take as needed.
3. The medication treats *only* the panic attacks. Once these are adequately controlled, you will need to enter Phase Two of treatment (graded reexposure) to deal with anticipatory anxiety and avoidance. In many cases this is best done with the help of a therapist familiar with behavioral techniques.
4. If MAO inhibitors are used, you must understand the dietary and medication restrictions and sign a consent form.
5. If alprazolam, lorazepam, or clonazepam are used, you must never abruptly discontinue it (medication reduction should be done gradually, generally 0.25 to 0.5 mg. per day per week).
6. If treated by antidepressants or MAOIs, it may take 2–4 weeks before you notice symptomatic changes.

*Social Phobias*

1. If medication is used (MAOI, SSRI, venlafaxine, or beta blockers), this must be accompanied by exposure (i.e., you must be willing to enter certain social situations and test out the water).
2. Psychotherapy is also indicated.

## Books to Recommend to Patients

1. Beckfield, D. (2004). *Master Your Panic,* Third Edition, Impact Publishers, San Luis Obispo, CA.
2. Bourne, E. (2003). *Coping with Anxiety.* New Harbinger Publications: Oakland.
3. Greist, J. H. and Jefferson, J. (2001). *Panic Disorder and Agoraphobia: A Guide,* Madison Institute of Medicine, Madison, Wisconsin.

# Chapter 5   Psychotic Disorders

## DIAGNOSIS

## Major Clinical Features and Differential Diagnosis

For practical purposes three major psychotic disorders are described: (1) schizophrenia (and schizophrenic-like disorders), (2) psychotic mood disorders, and (3) psychosis associated with neurological conditions.

Before discussing differential diagnosis, let's first briefly define *psychosis*. Psychosis is not an illness; it is a symptom associated with a number of disorders. The hallmark of psychosis is impaired reality testing (impaired ability to accurately perceive reality). The loss of contact with reality can take many forms: severe confusional states, delusions (bizarre, unrealistic thoughts), hallucinations, and marked impairment in judgement and reasoning. Having psychotic symptoms does not in itself imply a specific etiology; causes are varied. The three groups of psychotic disorders mentioned above are distinguished by the following characteristics:

1. *Schizophrenia*. Schizophrenia is generally a recurring illness; people diagnosed with schizophrenia are prone to repeated psychotic episodes. It is helpful to think about three types of schizophrenia:

   a. *Positive Symptom Schizophrenia*. This type of schizophrenia is also referred to as dopaminergic schizophrenia because of its presumed etiology: a hyperactive dopamine system. Positive systems are active, florid delusions and hallucinations; agitation and emotional dyscontrol. There are two subtypes:

      1. *Schizophreniform disorder* (Brief psychotic reaction). This disorder looks like schizophrenia but remits quicker and often does not recur.

      2. *Schizophrenia, per se.* This is a recurring or chronic disorder.

   b. *Negative Symptom Schizophrenia*. This is a neuro-developmental disorder. Negative symptoms include: flat or blunted affect, anhedonia (inability to experience pleasure), marked social aloofness/withdrawal, and the absence of florid delusions and hallucinations. Negative symptom schizophrenia tends to have an earlier and more insidious onset. As children, these people were often seen as odd and aloof.

2. *Psychotic Mood Disorders*. Both mania and depression can present with poor reality testing and other psychotic symptoms.

3. *Psychosis Associated with Neurological Conditions.* Many acute metabolic and toxic states can result in a delirium. Head injury occasionally produces transient psychotic behavior and a number of degenerative diseases (e.g., Alzheimer's) can produce periods of agitated confusion. Detailed description of psychopharmacologic treatment of various neurological conditions is beyond the scope of this book. However, it is very important to distinguish such conditions from schizophrenia and mood disorders. A brief mental status exam can be helpful. It should include a test of short-term memory, as well as tests for orientation and naming. Most neurologically based disorders that present with psychotic symptoms will also show gross impairment in recent/short-term memory; these abilities are relatively intact in schizophrenia. Damage to Wernicke's area (superior temporal lobe) can occasionally result in what looks like a schizophrenic reaction (language and thinking are grossly impaired). Wernicke's patients have a terrible time naming objects; people with schizophrenia and mood disorders do not. See the *Four Minute Neurological Exam* (in the MedMaster Series) for more hints on conducting a brief neurological exam. Figure 23 lists medical illnesses that may produce psychotic symptoms, and Figure 24 lists medications that may result in psychotic reactions.

*NOTE:* The treatment of mood disorders that present with psychotic symptoms primarily involves treating the depression (antidepressants or ECT) and adding antipsychotics to control the psychotic symptoms. Since much of this has been covered previously (Chapters 2 and 3), the focus of the following sections will be on treating schizophrenia.

## *Figure 23*

## COMMON DISEASES AND DISORDERS THAT MAY CAUSE PSYCHOSIS

- Addison's disease
- CNS infections
- CNS neoplasms
- CNS trauma
- Cushing's disease
- Delirium[1]
- Dementias[2]
- Folic acid deficiency
- Huntington's chorea
- Lewy body dementia[3]

- Multiple sclerosis
- Myxedema
- Pancreatitis
- Pellagra
- Pernicious anemia
- Porphyria
- Systemic lupus erythematosis
- Temporal lobe epilepsy
- Thyrotoxicosis

---

[1]Any number of toxic/metabolic states may result in delirium.
[2]Any number of dementing conditions (e.g., Alzheimer's disease) may result in psychotic symptoms.
[3]Caution: Only use quetiapine. Other antipsychotics can cause marked Parkinsonian symptoms.

*Figure 24*

## COMMON DRUGS THAT MAY CAUSE PSYCHOSIS

- Sympathomimetics (e.g., amphetamines, cocaine and "crack," a form of almost pure cocaine, many over-the-counter cold medications)
- Antiinflamatory drugs (e.g., steroids)
- Anticholinergic drugs (e.g., antiparkinsonian drugs)
- Hallucinogenic drugs (e.g., LSD)
- L-Dopa (in schizophrenic patients)

---

*NOTE:* Older persons are often on centrally acting drugs and have less ability to tolerate their toxic effects.


# Target Symptoms

It is helpful to subdivide schizophrenic symptoms into four categories: positive symptoms, disorganization symptoms, characterological traits, and negative symptoms. (See Figure 25.)


*Figure 25*

## SCHIZOPHRENIC SYMPTOMS

### POSITIVE SYMPTOMS

- Delusions and impaired thinking
- Hallucinations
- Confusion and impaired judgment
- Severe anxiety, agitation, and emotional dyscontrol

### NEGATIVE SYMPTOMS

- Flat or blunted affect
- Poverty of thought (i.e., few or no thoughts and concrete thinking)
- Emptiness and anhedonia (no joy)
- Psychomotor retardation/inactivity
- Blunting of perception (e.g., insensitivity to pain)

### DISORGANIZATION SYMPTOMS

- Incoherent speech
- Bizarre behavior
- Extreme confusion

### CHARACTEROLOGICAL TRAITS

- Social isolation and sense of alienation
- Low self-esteem
- Social skills deficits

# ANTIPSYCHOTIC MEDICATION

## When Do You Prescribe Antipsychotic Medication?

Although many general practitioners treat anxiety and depressive disorders, most patients presenting with psychotic symptoms should be referred to a psychiatrist. These patients are often hard to treat. Many psychotic patients can be treated on an outpatient basis; however, hospitalization may be necessary.

Antipsychotic medications (also referred to as neuroleptics or major tranquilizers) should be started when the early signs of psychosis appear, since many times a more florid psychotic episode can be averted with appropriate early intervention.

Positive symptoms and disorganization symptoms are the primary target symptoms for treatment by antipsychotic medications. Such drugs do little to affect characterological traits or negative symptoms (with some exceptions. See page 48).

## Choosing a Medication

All antipsychotic medications are equally effective in their ability to reduce positive symptoms. The choice of medication is dictated almost exclusively by the side effect profile. For a list of antipsychotic medications, see Figure 26.

Antipsychotic medications have five primary side effects which must be taken into consideration: sedation, anticholinergic (ACH), and extrapyramidal (EPS) effects, weight gain and metabolic effects.

Before choosing a medication, assess the patient's motor state. Psychotic reactions that present with marked agitation may require more sedating drugs. Use less sedating drugs for psychoses with pronounced psychomotor retardation and withdrawal. This is a general rule of thumb, but there are exceptions.

Consider anticholinergic and EPS side effects. The most common cause for relapse is poor compliance or premature discontinuation because of unpleasant side effects. The key to successful treatment rests on how well you handle side effects.

*Extrapyramidal Side Effects.* There are four classes of EPS:

1. *Parkinson-like Side Effects.* These include muscular rigidity, flat affect (mask-like facial expression), tremor, and bradykinesia (slowed motor responses). These symptoms need to be distinguished from the flat affect and withdrawal often seen as primary symptoms of schizophrenia. Parkinson-like side effects are often diminished by the administration of anticholinergic agents (e.g., benzotropine, trihexylphenidyl, or amantadine).

2. *Akathisia.* This is an uncontrolled sense of inner restlessness. Akathisia must be distinguished from anxiety. Often, a physician may mistake it for anxiety and increase the dose of antipsychotic, only to see a worsening of the restlessness. Akathisia can be partially alleviated by anticholinergic agents. Other

*Figure 26*

## ANTIPSYCHOTIC MEDICATIONS

| GENERIC | BRAND | DOSAGE RANGE[1] | SEDATION | EPS[2] | ACH EFFECTS[3] | EQUIVALENCE[4] |
|---|---|---|---|---|---|---|
| Low Potency | | | | | | |
| chlorpromazine | Thorazine | 50–1500 mg | High | + + | + + + + | 100 mg |
| thioridazine | Mellaril | 150–800 mg | High | + | + + + + + | 100 mg |
| clozapine* | Clozaril FazaClo | 300–900 mg | High | 0 | + + + + + | 50 mg |
| mesoridazine | Serentil | 50–500 mg | High | + | + + + + + | 50 mg |
| quetiapine* | Seroquel | 100–750 mg | High | + | + | 50 mg |
| High Potency | | | | | | |
| molindone | Moban | 20–225 mg | Low | + + + | + + + | 10 mg |
| perphenazine | Trilafon | 8–60 mg | Mid | + + + + | + + | 10 mg |
| loxapine | Loxitane | 50–250 mg | Low | + + + | + + | 10 mg |
| trifluoperazine | Stelazine | 10–40 mg | Low | + + + + | + + | 5 mg |
| fluphenazine | Prolixin[5] | 3–45 mg | Low | + + + + + | + + | 2 mg |
| thiothixene | Navane | 10–60 mg | Low | + + + + | + + | 5 mg |
| haloperidol | Haldol[5] | 2–40 mg | Low | + + + + + | + | 2 mg |
| olanzapine* | Zyprexa | 5–20 mg | Mid | + | + | 2 mg |
| pimozide | Orap | 1–10 mg | Low | + + + + + | + | 2 mg |
| risperidone* | Risperdal[5] | 2–10 mg | Low | + | + | 2 mg |
| ziprasidone* | Geodon | 60–160 mg | Low | + | + + | 10 mg |
| aripiprazole* | Abilify | 15–30 mg | Low | + | + | 2 mg |
| paliperidone* | Invega | 3–12 mg | Low | + | + | 1–2 mg |
| iloperidone* | Fanapt | 12–24 mg | mid | + | + + | 1–2 mg |
| asenapine* | Saphris | 10–20 mg | low | + | + | 1–2 mg |
| lurasidone | Latuda | 40–80 mg | low | + | 0 | 10 mg |

[1]Usual daily oral dosage

[2]Acute: Parkinson's dystonias, akathisia. Does not reflect risk for tardive dyskinesia. All neuroleptics may cause tardive dyskinesia, except clozapine.

[3]Anticholinergic Side Effects: dry mouth, constipation, urinary retention, and blurry vision.

[4]Dose required to achieve efficacy of 100 mg chlorpromazine.

[5]Available in time-released IM format.

* These medications are often referred to as "atypical" antipsychotics in that they have significantly less potential for causing extrapyramidal side effects than older-generation "typical" antipsychotics.

drugs, however, are often more successful. These include diphenhydramine, propranolol, or minor tranquilizers, such as lorazepam.

3. *Acute Dystonias.* These are muscle spasms and prolonged muscular contractions, usually of the head and neck. These can be resolved quickly with intramuscular anticholinergic agents, or treated prophylactically with oral anticholinergics.

4. *Tardive Dyskinesia (TD)*. TD is generally a late onset EPS. This is a very serious and often irreversible effect of antipsychotic medication treatment. It affects about one out of 25 people treated for a period of one year, and by seven years of continuous treatment, it affects one in four (in those treated with typical antipsychotics. TD rates are lower with newer, atypical drugs). Symptoms include involuntary sucking and smacking movements of the mouth and lips, and can include chorea in the trunk and extremities. Although various drugs have been used to reduce TD symptoms (e.g., baclofen, sodium valporate, lecithin, and benzodiazepines), there is no true cure. Treatment starts with stopping the medication. Initial worsening of the dyskinesia is expected, as the drug not only causes the syndrome but also tends to mask it. Be patient, for months if necessary, and TD will often remit. But control of severe psychosis usually outweighs the problem of TD. All patients receiving antipsychotics *must* sign an informed consent form which explains the risks of TD.

*Anticholinergic Side Effects*. Dry mouth, constipation, blurry vision, urinary hesitation, occasional delirium.

*Weight Gain*. Significant weight gain is a common problem with many of the antipsychotics (and may be a contributing factor increasing the risk of diabetes). Among the newer-generation antipsychotics two agents are recommended to avoid or minimize weight gain: ziprasidone (minimal weight gain) or aripiprazole (not associated with weight gain). It is not yet clear whether the decreased weight gain with these agents is associated with a lower risk of diabetes.

*Additional Side Effects*. Several potentially serious additional side affects can occur with antipsychotic medications, including agranulocytosis, possible prolongation of QTc interval (thioridazine, clozapine, mesoridazine, ziprasidone), impaired temperature regulations and thus increased risk of heat stroke or hypothermia, and neuroleptic malignant syndrome (a very rare syndrome that presents with fever, extrapyramidal rigidity, severe autonomic dysfunction and in some cases death). Increased risk of hyperglycemia, type II diabetes, weight gain, and elevations of triglycerides and cholesterol have been found in new generation, atypical antipsychotics, more commonly in clozapine and olanzapine. Risperidone, paliperidone, and quetiapine have a modest risk of these metabolic side effects. Thus patients treated with these drugs should be monitored carefully for these potential adverse effects. Such metabolic effects are rare in aripiprazole and ziprasidone. For these reasons, treatment of psychotic disorders is often more appropriately carried out by a psychiatrist.

## Prescribing Treatment and What to Expect

Antipsychotic medications are generally started at low to moderate doses and titrated up until there is reduction in the more disruptive aspects of the psychotic reaction, e.g., agitation. (*Note:* In the past, some clinicians have recommended "rapid neuroleptization," i.e., very high initial doses of neuroleptics. This treatment approach is controversial and not recommended.) Divided doses may be helpful initially; however, after a few days, a switch to a once-a-day bedtime dose is advisable.

Dosage ranges are extremely broad and vary considerably from patient to patient. In outpatient practice, an initial starting dose might be olanzapine 2.5 mg./day or quetiapine 100 mg./day. Inpatients are often treated at higher initial doses. See Figure 26 for dosage ranges. Antipsychotic medications must be taken each day.

Symptomatic improvement initially is seen as a decrease in arousal, emotional dyscontrol, and agitation. Poor reality testing, hallucinations, and disordered thinking may take much longer to respond. In many chronic schizophrenics, these latter symptoms may take a number of weeks to respond.

Assuming a good response, how long do you continue to treat? If the psychotic episode is a first episode, the rule of thumb is to decrease to a maintenance dose and continue to treat for one year. If the episode is a repeated episode, it will probably be best to treat for two to three years before a medication-free trial is initiated. Always, owing to the risk of TD, one should treat at the lowest possible dose that provides symptomatic relief.

# KEY POINTS TO COMMUNICATE TO PATIENTS

1. It is important to describe side effects to patients, especially akathisia. This side effect can be extremely unpleasant, yet often it is not spontaneously reported by patients. If it occurs and is not treated, this will greatly increase the risk of non-compliance, as well as increasing the patient's suffering. So tell patients, "You may notice an inner feeling of restlessness or nervousness. If you do, please tell me. Do not just discontinue the medication. Most side effects can be treated."

2. Schizophrenia is a relapsing disorder and it is extremely important to keep taking medication even if things seem fine. Premature discontinuation is the primary cause of relapse.

3. The total length of treatment is likely to be at least one year and often longer for more chronic schizophrenia.

4. Antipsychotic medications are not addictive.

5. You should avoid prolonged exposure to high temperatures and sunlight (some antipsychotics have photosensitivity as a side effect).

6. Avoid amphetamines, cocaine, and L-Dopa because these drugs almost always exacerbate psychoses.

7. You and your relatives need to know about and explain the risk of tardive dyskinesia (and sign appropriate consent forms.)

## Treatment-Resistant Schizophrenic Disorders

There are three main reasons why schizophrenic patients may not respond to antipsychotic medication:

1. *Poor compliance*. Often this is due to the unpleasant side effects. Many times patient education and proper medical management of side effects resolve the

## *Figure 27*

## DECISION TREE FOR DIAGNOSIS AND TREATMENT OF PSYCHOSIS

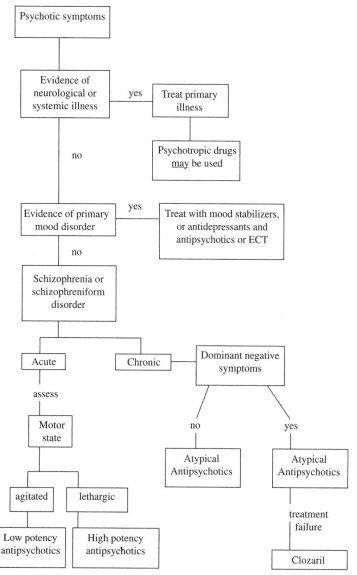

*Note:* In most cases due to favorable side effects, atypical antipsychotics are advised over the use of typical antipsychotics (unless long-acting IM antipsychotics are warranted).

problem. Sometimes, patients simply forget to take their medication. In such cases, treatment with time-released intramuscular forms of antipsychotics can be helpful (currently available for haloperidol and fluphenazine). Additionally, involving the family in treatment can significantly enhance compliance.

2. *Inadequate doses.* Blood levels can be monitored and doses increased as indicated.

3. Negative symptom schizophrenics may have a different underlying pathophysiology and often do not respond well to traditional antipsychotics. These patients are hard to treat.

Several, "atypical" antipsychotic medications have shown promise in treating the negative (as well as positive) symptoms of schizophrenia. The first is clozapine (brand name Clozaril). Clozapine became available in the United States in 1990. This medication is considered to be an atypical antipsychotic agent; its pharmacologic profile is different from other existing antipsychotics. The first important feature is that clinical trials show it to be effective in treating many schizophrenic patients who have failed to respond to standard antipsychotic drugs. This includes a number of patients that presented with negative symptoms (as well as other treatment-resistant schizophrenics). The second important and unique feature is the virtual lack of acute extrapyramidal symptoms and few reported cases of tardive dyskinesia. This medication does have two significant potential side effects: (1) The incidence of clozapine-induced agranulocytosis (a potentially fatal blood dyscrasia) is between 1 and 2%, as compared to the incidence seen in other antipsychotics (about 0.1%). This problem, however, is proving to be avoidable through a mandatory hematological monitoring program (weekly medication dispensing occurs only if the patient's white blood cell count is normal). Since implementing this program, there have been no fatalities in the 15 cases of clozapine-related agranulocytosis reported in the United States. If there is a low WBC count, medication is immediately discontinued and, to date, all such cases have been reversible. (2) A second troublesome side effect is a fairly high incidence of seizures (about 1–2% at low doses and 5% at higher doses). Despite these problematic features, clozapine appears to represent an important breakthrough in the management of otherwise treatment-resistant schizophrenic disorders.

The newest additions to the "atypical" list are aripiprazole, risperidone, olanzapine, quetiapine, paliperidone, and ziprasidone, providing additional options for treating both positive and negative psychotic symptoms with a much more benign side effect profile when compared to standard antipsychotics. These medications do not have the high incidence of agranulocytosis seen with clozapine.

## Common Treatment Errors to Avoid

- Akathisia (extreme inner sense of restlessness) is a very common side effect that is quite uncomfortable and a primary cause for patient-initiated discontinuation. Remarkably, many schizophrenic patients will not spontaneously complain of this side effect, but simply discontinue. It is therefore important to inquire specifically about the presence of akathisia during follow-up visits.

- Be especially watchful for early signs of tardive dyskinesia. Early signs can be elicited by having the patient lay his/her arms on lap while seated, extending the fingers in a relaxed, downward position over the knees. *Note:* Look for the presence of spontaneous, purposeless, jerking movements of the fingers.
- Antipsychotics often produce significant emotional blunting and apathy or Parkinsonian symptoms which may be mis-identified as negative symptoms (in such cases, raising the dose will likely exacerbate the side effects).

## Book to Recommend to Patients and Their Families

Torrey, E.F. (2001). *Surviving Schizophrenia: A Family Manual*, Harper and Row Publishers.

# Chapter 6   Miscellaneous Disorders

In this chapter we would like to briefly discuss six additional disorders for which psychotropic medications can be useful.

## OBSESSIVE-COMPULSIVE DISORDER

### Major Clinical Features

The major features of this disorder are recurring obsessions (persistent, intrusive, troublesome thoughts or impulses that are recognized by the patient as senseless) and/or compulsions (repetitive behaviors or rituals enacted in response to an obsession, e.g., repeatedly checking to see if doors are locked, compulsive hand washing, or counting). In order to meet the criteria for obsessive compulsive disorder, the obsessions and/or compulsions must create significant distress or be time consuming enough to interfere with normal routines.

### Medication Treatment

Treatments of choice include the use of serotinergic antidepressants (see below) often in combination with behavior therapy. Without behavior therapy, full relapse is likely with discontinuation. Thus, chronic medication treatment is generally necessary. Where most anxiety disorders generally respond to antidepressant treatments in 4–8 weeks, often progressive and gradual improvement in obsessive compulsive symptoms continue to be seen during the first 12 months of treatment. At about a year, generally a plateau is reached.

*Figure 28*

| NAME | | | | |
|---|---|---|---|---|
| Generic | Brand | Dose Range | Sedation | ACH Effects |
| clomipramine | Anafranil | 150–300 mg | Hi | Hi |
| fluoxetine | Prozac[1] | 20–80 mg | Low | None |
| sertraline | Zoloft[1] | 50–200 mg | Low | None |
| paroxetine | Paxil[1] | 20–50 mg | Low | Low |
| fluvoxamine | Luvox | 50–300 mg | Low | Low |
| citalopram | Celexa | 10–60 mg | Low | None |
| escitalopram | Lexapro | 5–20 mg | Low | None |
| vilazodone | Viibyrd | 10–40 mg | low | None |

[1]Often higher doses are required to control obsessive-compulsive symptoms than the doses generally used to treat depression.

# BORDERLINE PERSONALITY DISORDER

## Major Clinical Features

Borderline personality disorders constitute a very heterogeneous group of individuals that suffer from long-term emotional instability. As a group they are characterized by the following features: a pattern of chaotic, unstable relationships, extreme neediness, significant emotional lability, impulsiveness (e.g., self-mutilation, suicide attempts, substance abuse, very poor frustration tolerance, sexual promiscuity), anger control problems (e.g., pronounced irritability, temper tantrums, etc.), a tendency to develop significant bouts of anxiety and depression, and chronic feelings of emptiness. Some borderline patients can develop transient psychotic symptoms (that usually remit within hours to days). These patients are prone to a number of major psychiatric syndromes in addition to a very stable, chronic pattern of maladaptive functioning in life.

## Medication Treatment

Although there is increasing data to suggest an underlying biologic cause in many of these patients, it is generally felt that the basic disorder is an outgrowth of significant early, maladaptive psychological development (e.g., severe child neglect). Psychotropic medications do not treat the basic personality disorder, however, medications can be used to treat particular target symptoms.

Not all borderline patients are alike, and for treatment purposes, the following subgroups can be delineated to provide guidelines for choosing medications. The subgroups are defined by the presence of a dominant symptom picture. *Note:* Investigators to date have found that minor tranquilizers generally are not indicated in the treatment of borderline personality disorder. These patients often experience an increased degree of emotional dyscontrol/disinhibition with minor tranquilizers, and are at high risk for abusing such drugs.

*Figure 29*

| SUB-GROUPS | DRUGS OF CHOICE |
|---|---|
| 1. Impulsivity/Anger Control Problems | Serotonergic antidepressants, e.g., fluoxetine, sertraline. Omega 3 fatty acids: 1–2 grams qd |
| 2. Schizotypal (peculiar thinking, transient psychosis) | Low doses of antipsychotic medications, e.g., 2.5 mg olanzapine, 1 mg. risperidone |
| 3. Extreme sensitivity to rejection/ being alone | Serotonergic antidepressants, atypical antipsychotics |
| 4. Emotional instability | Lithium, divalproex, atypical antipsychotics |

# ATTENTION DEFICIT HYPERACTIVITY DISORDER

Attention deficit hyperactivity disorder (ADHD) affects 5% of children. It is now widely held that this disorder is largely due to a neurochemical disturbance (likely involving dysregulation of dopamine genetically transmitted in the frontal cortex).

Recent longitudinal/follow-up studies indicate that as many as 66% of ADHD children continue to exhibit symptoms well into adolescence and adult life, thus suggesting that potentially 2–3% of the adult population experience ADHD symptoms. The major symptoms of ADHD are outlined in Figure 30.

## *Figure 30*

## SYMPTOMS OF ADHD

- Impulsivity, e.g. acting before thinking, quick responses, poor judgment
- Difficulties in feeling motivated
- Impaired abilities for attention and concentration; distractibility
- Difficulties organizing tasks and activities
- Restlessness and "hyperactivity"
- Impaired emotional controls
- Associated features:
    Learning disabilities
    Low self-esteem

With age and maturation 33% of ADHD kids "grow out of it" and exhibit no ongoing symptoms. The remaining 66% tend to see a gradual reduction in restlessness and "hyperactivity" although other core ADHD symptoms remain.

ADHD kids and teenagers often encounter considerable social/peer rejection and academic failure. Self-esteem problems and frank clinical depression are not uncommon. Rates of substance abuse in *un*treated ADHD adolescents are high (probably best seen as an attempt to medicate-away feelings of sadness and inadequacy).

The discussion of pharmacologic treatment of ADHD with children and young teens is beyond the scope of this book (see Preston, O'Neal and Talaga, 2006). Older adolescent and adult ADHD clients can be very successfully treated with psychotropic medications (success rates approaching 90%).

The mainstay of pharmacologic treatment of ADHD is the use of stimulants (See Figure 31). Please note that the four fast-acting stimulants listed (methylphenidate, dexmethylphenidate, amphetamine, and dextroamphetamine) can become drugs of abuse in those predisposed to chemical dependency. Thus caution should be exercised in treating patients with a substance abuse history. (*Note:* Studies of ADHD